Praise for *Vegan Voices*

"*Vegan Voices* brings you the thoughts and experiences of the visionaries who have built this powerful movement. From ethics and activism to aesthetics and economics, it looks at all sides, charting an optimistic way forward for humans and for all the other animals with whom we share the planet."—**Neal D. Barnard**, MD, FACC, President, Physicians Committee for Responsible Medicine, Washington, DC

"As a vegan for forty-seven years, I appreciate *Vegan Voices* as a delightful and well-rounded holistic approach to veganism as a way of life as well as eating. I fully recommend this book to all levels of vegan readers. It points to veganism as a way to sanctify our eating. In each generation, we are given the medicine for healing that generation. Veganism is the medicine for healing this generation and also future generations. *Vegan Voices* gives a wonderful understanding of the vegan approach and understanding of life."—**Rabbi Gabriel Cousens**, MD, MD(H)

"There are as many reasons to be vegan as there are vegans, as this lovely anthology makes clear. So many of my heroes in one place—what a treat. Read it and be inspired."—**Bruce Friedrich**, Co-founder & Executive Director, The Good Food Institute

"If we are to have any hope of healing our damaged planet, it is clear that we must first rethink our relationship with animals. As *Vegan Voices* eloquently describes, for too long we've regarded the sentient beings with whom we share the world as mere things—commodities to be used for food, clothing, research, and entertainment. This is an important book that will serve as a call to action for every consumer to seriously consider the consequences of their dietary choices. *Vegan Voices* demonstrates that being vegan truly is a matter of life and death, and each one of us can make a difference."—**Mark Hawthorne**, author of *A Vegan Ethic: Embracing a Life of Kindness Toward All*

"Reading *Vegan Voices*, I found it fascinating to discover how others became enlightened, whether through their own observation, being taught by others, or through our subconscious with our 'mirror neurons' allowing empathy to not judge and misjudge other species. The variety of backgrounds presented here illustrates how we all can come together regardless of where we start. From philosophy professors to bodybuilders, it works for all! A 'Must Read!'"—**Ruth E. Heidrich**, PhD, author of *A Race for Life* and *Senior Fitness*

"*Vegan Voices* is a wonderful testament to the inspiring individuals around the world who are part of a growing paradigm shift towards more compassionate living."—**Sebastian Joy**, Founding President of ProVeg International

"This inspiring collection of essays presents the plight of animals and the activism in many forms meant to redeem our species by following an approach of live and let live. The volume seeks all attention from the ideal reader who with open heart and mind listens to the reasonable and passionate narrative experience of writers trying to convey the songs, the cries, and interests of our fellow animal friends from all different species."—**Anita Krajnc**, Founder, Animal Save Movement

"The beauty of this book is the self-realization that we ALL are inspiring changemakers!"—**Keegan Kuhn**, Co-director of *What The Health* and *Cowspiracy*

"Would you like to be radiant and vibrantly healthy? Do you want to experience vitality and joy throughout all your years? Would it matter to you if the most important steps you can take towards a long and healthy life also brought more compassion into the world, and also helped preserve our endangered ecosystems? That may sound fanciful, like it's too good to be true. But it isn't. It's the literal truth, as the essays in this book will show you with crystal clarity."—**John Robbins**, best-selling author, and President of Food Revolution Network

"Animals have voices, but humans don't speak their languages—so vegan voices speak for them. And this book allows everyone to tune in."
—**Ingrid Newkirk**, President and Founder of People for the Ethical Treatment of Animals (PETA)

"A beautifully inspiring and informative read for everyone who cares about animals. Dr. Joanne Kong has compiled an invaluable resource with unique experiences and wisdom from advocates across the globe, tapping into a broad range of topics. This just may be the inspiration that will spark your life's passion and ignite your sense of purpose in changing the world for the better."—**Jen Riley**, Director of Operations at Our Hen House

"Being vegan goes beyond what is at the end of your fork. As the accomplished authors of these inspiring essays illuminate, it also encompasses health, spirituality, environmentalism, compassion, kindness, and activism, coupled with a vital sense of unity, purpose, and consistency."
—**Jo Stepaniak**, MSEd, author of numerous groundbreaking books on vegan cuisine, health, and compassionate living

"This book offers inspiring insights into how animal activists became who they are. Discerning the most successful strategies for their vegan advocacy, the individuals in this book show that through a redirection of our personal and professional lives, we can create a world that works for all beings!"—**Veda Stram**, All-Creatures.org

VEGAN VOICES

Essays by Inspiring Changemakers

Dr. Joanne Kong
Editor

Foreword by
Victoria Moran

Lantern Publishing & Media ● Brooklyn, NY

2021
Lantern Publishing & Media
128 Second Place
Brooklyn, NY 11231
www.lanternpm.org

Cover design by Rebecca Moore
Book design by Emily Lavieri-Scull
Copy editing by Hanh Nguyen

Printed in the United States of America

Library of Congress Cataloging-in-Publication Data

Names: Kong, Joanne, 1957- editor.
Title: Vegan voices : essays by inspiring changemakers / Dr. Joanne Kong, editor ; with a foreword by Victoria Moran.
Description: Brooklyn, NY : Lantern Publishing & Media, 2021. | Includes bibliographical references.
Identifiers: LCCN 2021013008 (print) | LCCN 2021013009 (ebook) | ISBN 9781590566503 (paperback) | ISBN 9781590566510 (epub)
Subjects: LCSH: Veganism—Philosophy. | Raw foods. | Nutrition. | Diet—Moral and ethical aspects.
Classification: LCC TX392 .V424 2021 (print) | LCC TX392 (ebook) | DDC 613.2/622—dc23
LC record available at https://lccn.loc.gov/2021013008
LC ebook record available at https://lccn.loc.gov/2021013009

.

This book is dedicated to all animals needlessly exploited and killed,
and those around the world who serve as their voice.

Contents

About the Editor
About the Publisher

FOREWORD

Victoria Moran

Hope is important because it can make the present moment less difficult to bear.—Thich Nhat Hanh

This collection of essays is ostensibly about veganism, but veganism is about hope. In fact, there may be no hope without it.

Vegan living can propel to fruition the deepest yearnings of humanity—for freedom, health, self-actualization, spiritual growth. For an individual, living without harming—to the extent that it's possible—brings these visions within reach, and provides a boost of physical and psychic energy to bring them to fulfillment. Each person who contributed to this book illustrates in their essay how this has come about for them.

The bigger question, of course, is what life on Earth would look like if the vast majority of humans were vegan. Let's take this journey of hope together. For starters, the reduction in greenhouse gas emissions alone could change the future of life on this planet, perhaps ensuring that life would, in fact, endure for most species, our own included. Growing crops for human consumption instead of livestock feed would, when coupled with enlightened distribution, end hunger around the globe. Future pandemics would likely cease entirely, since almost every contagious scourge on record, from measles to (probably) COVID-19, came directly from human use and misuse of our animal brethren. Degenerative disease, also largely diet-related, would become much less of a burden on healthcare systems and on families with loved ones spending decades in decline.

And the cessation of human-caused misery in the animal world would be the most profound event in the ethical history of this planet. It would affect chickens, turkeys, and geese; pigs, cows, sheep, and goats;

and myriad kinds of fishes. It would liberate hunted animals, fur-bearers, and those wild beings whose rangeland humans claim for grazing cattle. The cages in laboratories would empty and their inmates—rats and mice, rabbits and guinea pigs, cats and dogs, and nonhuman primates—would no longer be subject to pain and death for someone else's knowledge, someone else's funding. Entertainment that enslaves animals would be universally deemed barbaric and would end without fanfare. And no more "pets" would be chained, ignored, abused, or abandoned.

As this healing revolution sweeps across nations, people could tackle remaining problems with renewed vigor. The fear and dread that keep the majority of caring humans trudging Eeyore-like beneath a gray cloud would lift. The sun would shine on Earth and all its inhabitants. Creativity would flourish. Peace would become inevitable, since the human family would be united as one kind and clever clan in the incredible web of livingkind.

It's a beautiful thought, right? But what if I've overshot? What if life can never be *that* good, or what if humans will never be *that* vegan? I'll take two-thirds. Heck, I'll take one-third. One-third of heaven on Earth makes for a reasonably heavenly Earth. And if we make that much progress, we'll make more.

As you read these essays, I invite you to look for synchronicities and serendipities, the unlikely occurrences that moved each writer forward on their journey to veganism, and those that took things from zero to sixty after this person went vegan. It seems to me that God or the Universe or the Force from *Star Wars* has determined that it is now time for this particular evolutionary leap to take place. Whatever the cause, you'll see in almost all of these engaging writings paths dotted with opportunities for travel, education, or a move that would change, well, just about everything. In other cases, it's a chance encounter with a person, book, film, or social media post that altered the course of a life, and enabled this individual to positively affect more lives.

That's another aspect of the hopefulness. For the boons of vegan living to come to us, we have only to start on this journey. And for that incredible, possible vegan world to take shape calls first for enough of us to take this journey. It's a grand adventure, to be sure, in which you'll experience hope and offer it—to the sanctuary pig you sponsor, your vegan grandchild, members of the plant-based Meetup group you start, even the amazing network of arteries inside your own body. Whether your vegan transition is overnight or over time, you're on the way to having your own vegan voice. The world is waiting to hear it.

INTRODUCTION

Dr. Joanne Kong

Veganism is a revolution of the heart, a call for a world of greater peace, health, and harmony created through expanding our circles of compassion. Interest in veganism as a mainstream movement that broadly touches many aspects of our lives continues to grow around the world. These aspects include health and wellbeing, sustainability, a desire to lessen the suffering of our kindred animals, and a reawakening of our deep capacities for kindness and empathy. I know you will be inspired by the writers in this book, who share a path and sense of purpose to create positive change in the world.

The motivations of those embarking on the vegan journey are highly individual, often deeply personal. Be it out of a desire to improve one's health, reduce the environmental devastation of animal agriculture, live in closer alignment with one's values, or address other issues such as social justice and ethics, such a motivation reflects a paradigm shift whereby one has begun to seriously question the underpinnings of a culture that has brought more and more harm to other beings, the natural world, and ourselves.

The awakening of new perceptions in regard to our lifestyle choices can begin in different ways. Some describe it as a light-bulb moment of sudden inspiration or realization. For others, a specific event or happening sparks an interest in veganism, or they become moved by a special connection with a particular animal. And for yet others, it is an awareness that grows over time.

My own path to veganism began in the early 1980s when, one day, my husband brought home a book titled *Animal Factories* by Jim Mason and Peter Singer. Little did I realize that this was a groundbreaking and controversial book, among the very first to expose the cruelty of factory farming. After reading the book, we resolved then and there to forever leave animals off our plates. In truth, it was one of the easiest decisions we had ever made. Yet, as I saw for the first time (black and white) photos of animals in these horrible industrial facilities, my mind kept turning to these questions: "Why had I never thought of this before?" and "How can I possibly continue to be a part of such immense suffering and violence?"

These questions are central to the purpose of this book, and have taken on increased importance in light of the connections between the coronavirus pandemic and humans' exploitation of animals. It is critical that such a global crisis be viewed not as a one-time occurrence, one which the world deals with then returns to normal. Rather, it is symptomatic of how society as a whole has lost its sense of balance with the natural world. Humankind has reached the point of inflicting the greatest damage upon the planet and its inhabitants, and we've been brought to a point of reckoning. We are awakening to the realization that many of the ways in which we live are unsustainable, and that we must move beyond an egocentric view of the world. Our collective thoughts and actions have profound consequences for the world around us, and our survivability will face greater and greater threats if we continue the false illusion that we can bend nature to our will.

Veganism is so significant because it addresses our sense of identity and the fundamental tenets of compassion. It is about truly living the Golden Rule and asking the defining question, "Do we see ourselves in all others?" It will be clear to you that the writers in this book have a common mission—to give voice to the voiceless, the tens of billions of innocent creatures who are needlessly killed every year. With these writers I share a passion for opening minds and hearts to seeing animals as kindred spirits, beings who share our capacities for emotion, cognition, socializing, caring, and having an interest in living. How can we promote peace, justice, empathy, and understanding in our world when we as a culture are complicit in the largest amount of suffering, destruction, death, and oppression taking place on our planet today?

The astounding cruelty inflicted upon nonhuman animals, whether through the food, research, entertainment, or clothing industry, is a reality hidden in plain sight. It is perhaps the greatest cognitive dissonance of our time. We know on some level that violence and death are inflicted on animals who are just as individual as our own pets, yet throughout most of society there persists an avoidance—even if at a subconscious level—of facing that reality. In addition, the economic and political power of the animal agriculture industry constantly normalizes animal exploitation as the status quo. As a result, within the foundations of our culture lies a tacit acceptance of force and violence used against others. Long-standing lifestyle habits easily become a source of security, stability and even validation, allowing the cruelty to continue. Many animal advocates would agree that in our efforts to educate others about the realities of factory farming, one of the most common responses is, "Don't tell me—I don't want to think about it!" Such reactions, in my view, are not about the shortcomings or insensitivities of others. Rather, these responses happen because our capacity to love is so great that we *want* to look away, to protectively distance ourselves from the discomfort and pain of seeing others suffer. Moving toward a culture of veganism is about "taking the blinders off," and breaking through the collective hardening and desensitization of our hearts that have resulted from thousands of years of animal domination. It's about ending our disconnection from the violence and death brought upon these innocent, sentient, vulnerable beings, and embracing and putting into action our innate empathy and compassion.

For many, becoming vegan is a transformational experience that improves their quality of health and day-to-day life, yet it is so much more. Going against the ingrained acceptance of superiority wielded against others, it's a courageous reimagining of the possibilities for a kinder, gentler world, one of greater equality and empathy among all living beings. Our vegan bravery is about many things—bringing ourselves to a full, conscious awakening to the horrific injustices inflicted upon nonhuman animals, opening ourselves to making changes in our lives that tie into our sense of identity and how we relate to kindred beings and the natural world, and living our ethical choices to lessen the suffering of others, even as we experience immense sadness, emotional pain, frustration, and despair in the face of a still mostly nonvegan world. In choosing a path that we feel to be right, we do so even if it means facing resistance or opposition from others, including family and friends.

To those of you who are new to veganism, I hope this book will open up new means of reflecting upon the many ways our lives take shape and touch others. Ultimately, the interest in and desire to adopt a plant-based diet go beyond just a lifestyle change, pointing to the power we have as individuals to shift humankind to a new, elevated level of compassion and caring. As Shankar Narayan, one of the contributors in this book, says, "Veganism is not a destiny; it's a journey." While the amazing individuals in this book have each found their own unique "vegan voices," their stories reflect life challenges that many of us share—improving our health and wellbeing, seeking happiness and fulfillment, exploring our values and sense of identity, finding where we "fit in" within society, and seeking meaning and purpose in our lives. The writers come from all around the world, with diverse roles as activists, educators, artists, writers, speakers, community organizers, entrepreneurs, sanctuary owners, health professionals, environmental advocates, and those who bear witness. And for those of us already actively promoting veganism, this book is a reminder that we are not alone; we can draw collective strength and motivation from a community of dedicated individuals who are laying the path for a more compassionate and inclusive world. I am deeply grateful to the writers whose essays fill this book, and continue to be inspired by their courage and passion as they work on behalf of animals. I would also like to express immense gratitude to Martin Rowe and Brian Normoyle of Lantern Publishing & Media for making this book project possible, and for the invaluable guidance they provided to make this book become a reality.

May your own journey be one of continuing personal transformation, as you embrace compassion toward all beings and fill your heart with the simple yet powerful truth that we are all connected.

SECTION ONE
Our Kindred Animals

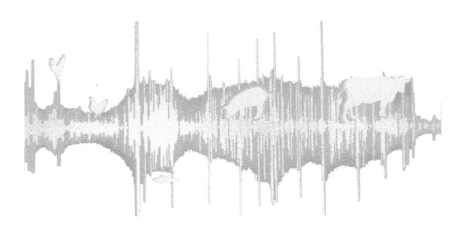

Laura Barlow

Activist, Educator, and President,
Rhode Island Vegan Awareness

Laura Barlow developed a passion for nature and animals at a young age. She spends her free time volunteering, running a nonprofit organization and taking care of her two rescue dogs. Her purpose in this world is to spread a message of love and compassion toward nature, animals, and humanity. Laura holds both a Master of Fine Arts and a Master of Education degree from Rhode Island College. She is certified in plant-based nutrition and pet therapy. Laura is a performing arts teacher in Providence, and currently resides in Warwick, Rhode Island.

Dogs for Dinner

It is the late 1990s. I am a typical teenager. This summer, I am earning spending money by working at the local supermarket. I stand behind the counter, staring at the clock. I count down the seconds. Finally, my shift is over. I make my way through the store, punch out at the time clock, and wait for my ride. At last, I arrive home. My dog greets me at the door with a kiss. I have a snack and head to my bedroom. I have something on my mind. I heard about veganism today at work and my curiosity is piqued. I wait for my dial-up Internet to load. Finally, I begin my research. My search takes me to a popular animal protection website. I click *play* on one of the many videos. This is the first time I see video footage from inside factory farms and slaughterhouses. I am devastated, to say the least.

The video is awful, but I cannot stop watching. I see piglets being slammed head-first on concrete floors. I see ducks having metal pipes shoved down their throats. I watch as animals are crammed into tiny, filthy cages. My jaw drops as I observe chicks being ground up alive.

My heart races as I view animals being castrated and having their tails chopped off without painkillers. I watch in horror as animals are dehorned and debeaked. I hear animals screaming out in pain. I feel my heart breaking. I can't fight back my tears. Many of my beliefs are being shattered. I have so many questions. How is this legal? Why won't anyone stop this? Why is this happening? What can I do to help?

As a self-proclaimed animal lover, I am outraged. I love animals, especially dogs. I look over at my dog. I love everything about him. I love his soft ears, four paws, cold nose, and unique personality. My mind races. I begin to make an important connection between farmed animals and my pets. Suddenly, I realize that they are kindred animals. They all have beating hearts. They all have unique personalities. I can see that there are differences between animals, but at this moment it is the similarities that matter.

Making this connection has a profound impact on me. I am suddenly forced to take a deep look at myself. Prior to this point in my life, I wasn't acting like a person who loved all animals. I was acting in a way that showed love for some animals and not others. I begin to understand that you cannot eat a being you love. You cannot support cruelty toward animals and claim to love them. I spend hours doing research that evening before going to bed. When I wake up the next morning, *I am a vegan.* For the first time in my life, my actions and ethics align. I feel peace and love in my heart for all animals.

Many things changed for me that day. It was especially upsetting when I realized that I had been contributing to the suffering of animals. I was consuming the products of their suffering. Prior to that day, I was like many people who claim to be against animal cruelty while simultaneously contributing to it. I was claiming to love animals while at the same moment eating them.

There was a lot of guilt involved in realizing that my actions were causing harm to animals. I wish that I had gone vegan sooner, but came to understand that I was not a bad person before going vegan. I just had not made that important connection, yet I feel very blessed that I made the connection at a young age. I also know that it is never too late to make a positive difference. Anyone can decide to go vegan and stop contributing to animal cruelty at any time and that is beautiful.

Throughout the years, I have watched many videos and films that show cruelty to animals. Despite being difficult to watch, these films are necessary. In recent years, a great deal of attention has been focused on dog meat farms. Dogs on meat farms are crammed into tiny, filthy cages. These dogs may be killed by electrocution, blunt force, hanging, or even by being boiled alive. My heart breaks when I see these images and videos. The dogs look broken and hopeless, and their eyes reveal a life of pain and suffering. In their eyes, I see all animals whose suffering is for human consumption and profit. All of these animals experience pain, suffering, and fear. They all quiver before their death. The truth is that all animals want to live.

It is now 2020 and I am in my late thirties. I can proudly say that I love all animals. My love for animals is reflected through my vegan lifestyle and activism. I do everything I can not to contribute to their suffering. Going vegan is the best decision I have ever made. I also run a nonprofit organization, Rhode Island Vegan Awareness, that is dedicated to advocating veganism for a more peaceful and just world for all life.

I write this essay during the height of a pandemic. The virus has an animal origin, and it is believed that its early spread may have been linked to a seafood market that also killed and sold live animals for human consumption. Slaughterhouses and factory farms are hell on Earth for animals. It is important to note that the harm doesn't stop there. Our planet and all who inhabit her are suffering as a result of our dangerous, unhealthy, and damaging relationship to animals.

Baxter and Mama Belle are sleeping nearby. They are both rescue dogs. Mama Belle is blind and was rescued from the streets of Egypt. Baxter came from an Atlanta rescue. On this rainy day in December, I am very thankful for them. They are safe and loved. I wish all animals could feel this way. I long for the day when all animals will live in peace. I know many people are outraged at the idea of having dogs for dinner. I hope they will make the connection that I did. I dream of a world in which all people will be outraged at the idea of having any animal for dinner.

EMILY MORAN BARWICK

Activist, Educator, International Speaker, Writer, Artist

Emily Moran Barwick was born with a fierce sense of justice. From authoring essays on the experiences of children in the foster care system at six to educating door-to-door about endangered species at seven, Emily's advocacy and activism took root at a very early age. After completing her Master of Fine Arts, Emily founded Bite Size Vegan, providing free resources and information on issues impacting health, our planet, society, and the lives of sentient beings. Communication has never come easily to Emily—an Autistic—but she credits her Autism for her deep and empathetic connection with nonhuman animals, and believes that by seeing the world differently, she's better able to help others begin to think differently.

THE HARM OF "HUMANE"

In September 2008, an undercover video documenting routine abuse at an Iowa pig-breeding facility made international news.[1] The footage and investigators' notes[2] captured workers kicking and beating pregnant pigs with metal objects and sexually violating them with metal rods; they were also shown cutting off the tails and tearing out the testicles of piglets without anesthetic, and slamming sick or deformed piglets against the ground, leaving them to die slowly, piled on top of one another in giant bins.

While these acts of cruelty were exposed by vegan activists, the egregiousness of the abuse sparked outrage from meat-eating consumers. Hormel, the food company supplied by the farm, received over ten thousand calls in two days.[3] In the wire report issued by the Associated Press, a Hormel spokesperson called the abuses "completely unacceptable"; the farm's owner emphasized, "We condemn these types of acts," calling them "completely intolerable, reprehensible," and vowed to "investigate and initiate corrective action immediately."[4]

Anyone reading the report would be left with the impression that this was an isolated incident of overt cruelty or—at the very worst—a regular occurrence isolated to large factory farms. Amidst the catalogued horrors, the troubling implication of a single sentence was easily overlooked; following the description of the workers' treatment of piglets, the report stated: "Temple Grandin, a leading animal welfare expert who serves as a consultant to the livestock industry, said that *while those are standard industry practices*, the treatment of the sows on the video was far from it. 'This is atrocious animal abuse,' Grandin said" (Associated Press 2008, emphasis added).

To be clear, the treatment of the mother pigs was what Grandin deemed "atrocious animal abuse"; the acts she waved away as "standard industry practices" were the unanesthetized mutilation of newborn piglets and the brutal—and ineffective—slamming of "defective" piglets against the concrete floor. She was not wrong: not only are these practices legal, they are government-sanctioned methods within—but not exclusive to—the United States,[5] Canada,[6] and the European Union.[7]

Ask yourself—were you to have watched that video, heard the piercing screams of the mother pigs and their babies, would you have spotted the difference between the "atrocious animal abuse" and "standard industry practices"?

Operating on Faith

Most people have faith—or assume—that regulations protect animals in our food industries.[8] Consumer concern over animal welfare has long been on the rise, with more "humane," "free-range," and "cage-free" options available than ever before.

Given that you're reading this book, chances are you, too, have concerns, and if you're anything like the majority of consumers, you're not sure what to believe.[9] Most people possess little to no knowledge of where their food comes from and how the individuals they consume were treated.[10] This isn't due to a lack of intelligence. This information is deliberately difficult to find; and even then, it's couched in euphemisms and dense legal language—inaccessible by design.

Which has to make you wonder—if there's really nothing wrong with how we breed, raise, and kill the animals we eat, why make such an effort?

The Realities of Regulations

In 2007, in a historical move, the European Union declared nonhuman animals legally sentient—deserving freedom from hunger, thirst, discomfort, pain, injury, disease, fear, distress, and mental suffering.[11] Having recognized animals' capacity to feel the same emotions and sensations as we do, the EU proceeded to draft landmark legislation for their humane treatment. The resulting Council Regulation[12] was—and is—viewed as a victory for animals. For those of us in countries without regulations, it's natural to think that the systematic abuse of farmed animals results—at least in large part—from the total lack of oversight.

In the United States, for example, there are *no federal laws* governing the treatment of animals in our food industry.[13] The Animal Welfare Act of 1966,[14] like so many welfare acts around the world, excludes animals raised for food—as do the majority of state anti-cruelty regulations.[15] Many US activists and organizations stress the need for regulations to end such atrocities as the routine mutilation without anesthetic, the maceration (grinding up) of male chicks in the egg industry, and the blunt-force "euthanasia" of piglets captured in the Iowa video—often pointing to the EU as a shining example.

However, within the EU legislation and supplemental documents, those *very same atrocities* are not decried but *codified.* So instead of male baby chicks being ground up alive because there are no regulations to stop it, they are ground up alive because regulations declare it the preferred method for male chick disposal. There are even detailed specifications for blade speed and sharpness to avoid "gumming up" the works.[16] The European Commission estimates that the EU kills 330 million chicks every year,[17] with global estimates at 3.2 billion.[18]

This isn't a barbaric practice isolated to corrupt, abusive facilities or industrialized factory farms. Grinding up live babies is a welfare regulation—a *worldwide* "standard practice."

Yet every time an undercover video is released documenting chicks falling off a conveyor belt into a grinder, people are appalled. They assume—as with the Iowa footage—that it's an isolated incident of extreme cruelty and they continue to eat eggs, confident they're not supporting such brutality.

Down to the Dollar

We'd like to think that humane regulations are driven by what's best for the animals. But the animal products industries are, after all, industries; they are profit-driven. Take the European Union legislation specifying maceration for male chick "disposal." A preliminary report found that while gassing the estimated "335 million day-old male chicks" killed in the EU annually would cost 1,665,000 euros, the cost of using "rotating or whirling knives which are mincing the chicks in a split second . . . can be considered not to be substantial."[19]

The decision had nothing to do with what was most humane—it was simply a matter of what was cheapest.

What's in a Label?

It's no surprise that humane food labels have gained a stronghold. To the vegan afraid of coming across as militant, they provide a less intimidating suggestion to offer the veg-curious; to activists fighting for animal liberation, they give the possibility of better living conditions for animals—progress toward the ultimate goal; and to the nonvegan, they offer a way to keep eating animals but feel good about it.

Unfortunately, the only comfort humane labels bring is to our conscience. "Cage-free" is meaningless for chickens raised for meat; they are never raised in cages as it is. In the egg industry, "cage-free" indicates that hens are not housed in battery cages. However, they may still be raised in overly crowded sheds, and "cage-free" hens have been shown to have *double the mortality rate* of battery-caged hens.[20]

In the United States, the only specification for "free-range" is that the animal "has been allowed access to the outside."[21] There are no standards for the amount of time outside, or the size and nature of the outside area. Facility inspections are not required for "cage-free" and "free-range" claims.[22]

Many labels like "humanely raised," "humanely treated," and "raised with care" lack any formalized meaning.[23] Producers are left to define *their own understanding* of what the terms mean.[24]

How "Humane" Harms

It may sound odd coming from an animal rights activist, but I find that humane labels and regulations are often detrimental to animals. Welfare regulations are designed to spare animals any "unnecessary" suffering—the unspoken implication being that some suffering is necessary when it benefits humans.

Still, even if animal liberation is the ultimate goal, isn't there value in improving the conditions of those currently in our systems of exploitation? While there is validity in this position, I find it vital to take an honest look at what welfare regulations *actually mean for the beings they are designed to protect.*

In the egg industry, the majority of the world's more than seven billion layer hens[25] spend their abbreviated lives in cramped battery cages. The European Union, once again at the forefront of animal welfare, issued a groundbreaking directive in 1999, banning "barren battery cages" by 2012.[26] From the media headlines, you'd be left with the impression that EU hens would be cage-free. In reality, the directive merely replaced *barren* battery cages with *"enriched"*—meaning furnished—battery cages. Reports extolled how hens would now each be afforded 750 cm^2, neglecting the clarification that only 600 cm^2 would be usable due to "furnishings." Understanding the true impotence of this legislation makes its pathetic implementation all the more baffling. By 2012, thirteen member states had failed to comply with the ban.[27] These thirteen countries had had *over twelve years* to grant laying hens *less than a single playing card of additional space.*

But as the media celebrated the victory for animal welfare, the public ate even more eggs—reassured by their higher standards—and the individuals this entire charade was supposed to be for remained just as exploited. This is how "humane" harms.

The execution of the barren battery cage ban is far from the only failing. In 2001, the EU outlawed gestation crates—single-sow enclosures constructed of metal bars and hard flooring in which mother pigs are confined during their pregnancies. As always, the ban came with ample fine-print exceptions, and over a decade for implementation. Twelve years later, nine member states had still failed to comply with the ban.[28]

Several of the member states that failed to implement the battery cage ban and/or the gestation crate ban are rated amongst the best countries in the world when it comes to animal welfare.[29]

The Bottom Line

Underneath the convoluted legislation and industry propaganda, humane concepts are based on a faulty premise: that there is a compassionate way to enslave, violate, mutilate, and kill. Even if we imagine an idealized small farm where animals are given ample space outdoors, with their every need cared for, there would still come a time when their life is cut short. Now, imagine in their place a beloved family pet—would it be acceptable to end *their* life? What if you were guaranteed that they wouldn't feel a thing, that it would be quick and humane?

What is the difference between our pets and the sentient beings in the food industry? Do they not also feel pain and fear? When a mother cow in the dairy industry cries out for her calf—taken from her so she will produce more milk for humans—is that not a mother grieving? When she is sexually violated yet again, and made to undergo yet another pregnancy and give birth to yet another child who will yet again be taken—how can that not take an emotional and physical toll? There's a reason dairy cows' bodies generally give out at around age four to five, despite their natural life span of twenty years or more.[30]

Applying such emotionality to nonhuman animals is often criticized as anthropomorphic—an objection that illustrates the contradiction of humane concepts. Humane regulations are an inherent admission of animals' ability to suffer and feel pain. How can we claim that our animals are healthy and happy, then deny that they possess these capacities when asked to see from their perspective? We cannot have it both ways.

This is how profoundly illogical our thinking is when it comes to animals. Knowing better but doing wrong anyway is worse than having no knowledge. Yet we have the audacity to hold on high the legislative recognition of nonhuman sentience as a giant step forward for the rights of animals, as if systematically exploiting individuals with fully admitted knowledge and comprehension of their capacity to suffer were something to commend.

We campaign for regulations and wait over a decade for the smallest advances when all the while there is another option entirely. One that we don't have to manipulate our values to justify. One that we don't have to couch in euphemisms or bury beneath dense legislation. One that allows us to finally align our actions with our values.

You have a choice. You decide whether you want to continue to have others kill for you. You decide whether you want to continue consuming death, terror, and heartbreak—whitewashed as humane. You decide. My hope is you'll decide to go vegan.

KATINA CZYCZELIS

Business Manager, Musician, Activist, Writer, Healer

Katina Czyczelis graduated from the University of Adelaide with a First Class Honours Bachelor of Law degree and practiced as a barrister and solicitor until she gave the law up to have a family. She later graduated from the University of Adelaide with a Bachelor of Music Performance degree, performing, teaching, and writing about her instrument. She is currently employed as a general manager in the hospitality industry. Being a vegan of many years, and through speaking out and writing, Katina has dedicated herself to the life, freedom, and happiness of all animals on Earth.

MIGHT DOES NOT MAKE RIGHT

We have no right to use and enslave other living beings. Might does not make right. Past practice and culture do not make right. What is right is based on principles. These are the principles of ethics, morality, and justice. While a man may have the might to overtake and rape a woman, does this give him the right to do so? The answer is, "Absolutely not." Similarly, an adult may have the might to abuse a child, yet does this give the adult the right to do so? Again, the answer is, resoundingly, "Absolutely not."

So ethics, morality, and justice tell us that might does not make right, yet how do humans justify the use, enslavement, genetic manipulation, commodification, mutilation, objectification, killing, and consuming of sentient beings on this earth? The honest answer is we cannot, but we have tried to do so using any excuse and reasoning that we, as the wielders of power, can use. These excuses include religious invention, an insidious and grotesque way to justify violence as a way to condone and suit humans' practices and desires. And cultural practices are used to justify continuing insupportable barbarism in a time when there is no need for such practices to continue. Discrimination based on species (speciesism) is used to justify the inferiority of—and our dominion over—nonhuman beings. This is a foul and baseless line of reasoning, similar to discrimination and discriminatory actions based on color, race, or gender in the human species. Then there is the excuse of ownership, the result of the commodification of sentient living beings, which should be an affront and a perversion to any civilized mind. There are also people who simply do not care, and people who just want to satisfy their wants. For most of the world's population, in this day and age, there is absolutely no need to use or consume animals or animal products. The practice of doing so is due to the power of vested interest, habit, and selfishness.

We alone have the power and ability to choose what we consume, wear, or participate in. This factor of choice brings up questions of ethics and morality, and requires us to examine our reasoning in relation to ethical principles. Who are we as a species if we ignore these principles in order to sustain the selfish choices we make? Who are we as a species if we ignore the suffering, the cries, the needs, and the desire for happiness and peace of all the sentient beings of this earth? Who are we? Objective evidence shows that on the whole, we have been a selfish, cruel, and violent species, able to ignore, cause, profit from, and even enjoy the suffering of other living beings. We make up twisted excuses, embracing beliefs—not facts—to suit our desires.

What is it about the human who refuses to acknowledge that animals of nonhuman species also want to be free, happy, and comfortable, to love their families and just be in peace, rather than being enslaved, caged, farmed, killed, skinned, and used as entertainment or for pleasure? Why do some humans become angry, hateful, and violent toward those who want happiness for all beings? Most people are so indoctrinated with the present paradigm that they cannot see the lies they are supporting and believing; they cannot see the reality of what they are responsible for. That reality is a horror, a nightmare, a travesty, and an abomination.

Please watch documentaries such as *Cowspiracy, Speciesism: The Movie, Blackfish, Dominion, What the Health, Forks Over Knives, The Game*

Changers, The Path of the Horse, Before the Flood, Food Choices, Food, Inc., and *Earthlings.* The last is not pleasant to view, but if you realize the cruel reality of what is shown, how can you continue to consume animal products?

There is no excuse for ignorance at this time on Earth. The use of animals for food, experiments, apparel, and pleasure is damaging the planet severely, causing desertification on land and creating dead zones in the sea, destroying and polluting natural habitats, and being the main driver of the mass extinction of wildlife we are now seeing. The use of animals is, and has always been, the main cause of disease and illness in animals and humans, including the current COVID-19 pandemic. Most people have no idea that even the common flu was caused by animal farming.

Overall, compared to vegans, those who consume animal products are more susceptible to disease and conditions that require medications. Those who consume whole-food plant-based diets are in fact among the healthiest and longest-living. It has been shown that those who fully adopt a plant-based diet are able to alleviate or even heal chronic diseases.

Being vegan goes beyond just what we put into our stomachs. It extends to a rejection of the whole paradigm of using other living beings for our own selfish purposes. It extends to a recognition of what we are actually doing to other sentient beings. What makes it absolutely criminal is that we do these things to nonhuman beings not because we have to but simply because we can, and we choose not to end it. Everything is energy, and what we consume becomes a part of us, even at the subatomic and vibratory levels. Physicists have told us that energy does not disappear—it continues on, extending, shifting, moving, but it is not destroyed. So when we condone, participate in, or consume products of violence, slavery, denial, torture, or selfishness, the same degree of violence as that inflicted upon the nonhuman being is returned to us in one way or another. The energies of what we consume can manifest within us, whether as disease or depression. Everything is a product of vibration and energy. Everything vibrates into form and matter.

Unbiased studies and research show that consumption of animal products is linked to diseases such as cancers and cardiovascular disorders. Red meat is classified under Group 2 as a probable carcinogen. Animal flesh is now shown to contribute to aging. Dairy products are highly inflammatory and linked to various cancers and even osteoporosis. Eggs are also linked to various cancers as well as heart disease. It is now scientifically established that while we may obtain nutrients from animal products, we are also bringing disease upon our bodies from other substances they contain.

Vegans obtain necessary nutrients directly from plants, without the toxins, inflammatory agents, and cancer-causing chemicals found in animal products. In fact, through studies of human biology, physiology, anatomy, and digestion, it has been shown that humans actually evolved as plant eaters, able to obtain and manufacture what we need from the plant world. While our bodies may be able to tolerate some level of animal product consumption, humans essentially thrive on a whole-food plant-based diet. The whole-food plant-based diet has been shown to lengthen lifespan, improve human health, and even help with depression and emotional wellbeing. Please look up the groundbreaking work of Nobel Prize–winning geneticist Elizabeth Blackburn and read her book *The Telomere Effect*. Her work proves the longevity-promoting properties of a whole-food plant-based diet and the life-shortening properties of animal product consumption.

The fact is: for every single animal product or use of animals for textiles, food, plastics, technology, or testing, we can choose the ethical, plant-based alternative. The continued use of animal products in this day and age is destructive, backwards, ignorant, selfish, criminal, negligent, and an atrocity for how much suffering it causes. There is no such thing as sustainable meat. There is no such thing as ethical or kind meat, eggs, dairy, or other animal products. All such labels are lies. These words are used to make people feel better about their choices. Ultimately, I think most people *do* care but really choose not to look closely enough at their choices.

Nonhuman animals have so much in common with us. They have a central nervous system, digestive system, thought system, brain, and mind. They breathe, think, love, suffer, and feel pain, just as we do. Like us, they want to be happy and free to live their lives. We are more like nonhuman animals than we are different from them. Yet we enslave them, keeping them in herds and in cages, small spaces, zoos, and factory farms. We mutilate them to suit our purposes. We debeak and dehorn them. We mutate them into grotesque new breeds so that they grow more flesh or huge mammary glands to produce more milk. Hens are forced to lay eggs daily instead of a few times a year as they would naturally do in the wild. We trap them, skin them alive, and murder them. We take away their children, and deny them family and life. We masturbate males by the millions for their semen and repeatedly inseminate females, forcing them to give birth to more and more babies who are subsequently tortured, murdered, gassed, boiled, or burned alive. There is nothing ethical about that chicken flesh or glass of milk, as both were obtained through animal slavery and violence; both involve cruelty you would never want to experience yourself.

The animals commonly used for food, such as pigs, chickens, and turkeys, have been scientifically assessed to be as aware and intelligent as cats, dogs, parrots, and other beloved companion animals. Pigs, for example, are regarded as one of the most intelligent animals on Earth, yet are one of the most abused. It is time we face and act upon these scientific facts instead of accepting the misinformation spread by those who harm and commodify animals for their selfish needs.

We have laws recognizing that slavery, rape, mutilation, murder, and violence are wrong. There is no valid ethical reason to exclude nonhuman sentient beings from this protection. The distinction between the animals we exploit and those we don't is artificial and arbitrary, created to suit human, cultural desires and not based at all on morality or ethics. The intrinsic nature of the violence is not lessened just because it is committed against another species. The taking of a life of a being who doesn't want to die is murder. The act of enslavement constitutes slavery, regardless of the species of the one being enslaved. The perpetrated crime is felt in all its violence by the innocent being; it is always committed against his or her will. Animals are sentient individuals. That they are not of the human species does not take away their sentience or their desire to be happy and free. We must change what we are doing. Unlike the other animals of this earth, we have a choice. We must choose wisely and ethically, not out of cultural bias, self-interest, or ignorance.

Only *you* can change this violent and unethical paradigm—one based on lies, ignorance, cultural and religious pressure, and greed. Only with your choice to go vegan can we bring about the massive change needed to take away the violence we have been committing for so long against innocent, sentient beings of the earth. Only with this choice can we bring greater harmony, peace, and health, environmental prosperity, and the safety of wildlife back to Earth. What we do and give out is always returned to us—in one way or another.

Being vegan is the most profound and effective thing one can do in order to halt the present destruction on Earth. It is time to end animal slavery and the commodification of sentient beings. We can go vegan—and meet the ethical challenges of our times.

Animals are our friends if we only let that be possible.

Their hearts cry out to us. It is up to us to open up to their calls and pleas.

Let me ask you—what if it were *you* in their place?

KAREN DAVIS, PHD

President and Founder, United Poultry Concerns

Karen Davis, PhD, is the president and founder of United Poultry Concerns, a nonprofit organization that promotes the compassionate and respectful treatment of domestic fowl and operates a sanctuary for chickens in Virginia. Having been inducted into the National Animal Rights Hall of Fame "for outstanding contributions to animal liberation," Karen is the author of numerous books, essays, articles, and campaigns. Her latest book is *For the Birds: From Exploitation to Liberation: Essays on Chickens, Turkeys, and Other Domesticated Fowl* (Lantern, 2019).

WITH HEART AND VOICE:
WILL BIRDS SING OR WILL THEY BE SILENT?

In "Chickenomics—How Chicken Became the Rich World's Most Popular Meat," *The Economist* reported on January 19, 2019 that "the total mass of farmed chickens exceeds that of all other birds on the planet combined."[31] This startling statistic comprises 1) the unimaginable number and size of chickens suffering for food worldwide and 2) the disappearance of wild birds from the world.[32] As the prison population of chickens grows, the number of birds living free declines. The dwindling population of free birds includes the chicken's tropical forest ancestor and wild relative—the jungle fowl—whose habitat is being destroyed acre by acre, in part to grow soybeans for industrialized chickens.

In *Silent Spring*, Rachel Carson opens Chapter 8, "And No Birds Sing," with the observation that over increasingly large areas of the United States, spring now comes unheralded by the return of the birds, and the early mornings are strangely silent whereas once they were filled with the beauty of bird song. This sudden silencing of the song of birds, this obliteration of the color and beauty and interest they lend to our world, have come about swiftly, insidiously, and unnoticed by those whose communities are as yet unaffected.[33]

Silent Spring documents the effects of industrial chemicals on the planet and the reckless and careless conduct of human beings, of which this chemical catastrophe is a prime example. When the book first appeared in 1962, it was ridiculed and dismissed by those with corporate interests, but even after *Silent Spring* was hailed—grudgingly or gratefully—for its accuracy and justifiable urgency, little changed. Half a century later, wild animals are being harmed and killed every day by pharmaceutical waste, plastics, poisons, and the aggregating crises of climate change.[34]

Even so, more taxpayer dollars will probably be spent on trips to Mars and the moon than will ever be spent caring for the earth and its creatures. Recently, a cable news show host rhapsodized over a renovated space program. Listening, I wondered: If he knew how his fellow Earthling chickens are mired in misery and filth in metal sheds that look like they came from outer space for his food, would he care?

Something I learned about chickens when I started knowing them decades ago is how vocally charged they are from morning to night. All day long, I hear their voices outside, ringing and singing. Since we built our predator-proof outdoor aviary in 2014 so that our roosters and hens could perch safely in the bushes and trees if they liked, I have felt the true sense of their vocal exuberance and how utterly their voices express their vitality. The comical commotion each evening as they rustle around in the branches and leaves before settling down for the night evokes the tropical forest in which they evolved and the primal chords in the heart of each bird.

By contrast, if you open the door of a Tyson or Perdue chicken house after the newborns have been there for a week or so, you will not hear a peep or a rustle. If you enter a facility where hens have been caged for eggs for a few months, the sound of silence will strike you more forcibly than commotion. Of all the indicators of their suffering, the sound of thousands of chickens together, mute and unmoving, is the eeriest, most audible signal that something is wrong.

Some will argue that these chickens, having no basis for comparison, cannot know that their lives are desolate. We might as well use this plea to absolve ourselves of responsibility toward anyone in the world whom we decide, because they have never known anything but misery, "cannot know that their lives are desolate."

As a matter of fact, desolate individuals of all species *do* know, because knowing is an organic process far deeper than words and concepts can express. Every bodily cell is a repository of experiences, including memory and expectation, as elements of a particular moment in the life of that particular cell. The sorrows deep in a creature's eyes, the sound of a bird's unnatural silence and moaning tones of woe, tell us a whole lot about what they "know."

The idea that human beings cannot logically recognize suffering in a chicken, or draw meaningful conclusions about how we would react to the conditions in which a caged bird lives, is unfounded. Our capacity for empathy and understanding is grounded in the fact of human evolutionary continuity with other creatures, which enables us to recognize and infer in those creatures experiences similar to our own.

As the veterinary scholar Michael W. Fox observes, freedom and wellbeing "are more than intellectual concepts. They are a subjective aspect of being, not exclusive to humanity, but inclusive of all life. This is not an anthropomorphic claim. It is logically probable and empirically verifiable."[35]

This being so, there is the further presumption that forcibly confining chickens in environments that reflect aspects of human nature that birds do not share means that they suffer more than we know, in ways we can scarcely imagine. If chickens preferred being packed together, cut off from the outside world, then we would not need intensive confinement facilities and mutilations such as debeaking, since they would voluntarily come together, live cordially, and save us money. The egg industry thinks nothing of claiming that a mutilated hen in a cage is "happy," "content," and "singing," yet will turn around and try to intimidate you with accusations of "anthropomorphism" if you logically insist that the mute or crying hen with the sunken or frantic eyes is miserable.

In *Silent Spring*, Rachel Carson writes: "From all over the world come echoes of the peril that faces birds in our modern world."[36] I hope that her elegiac plea for attention and action for the birds included a thought for the chickens who, at that very time, in the 1960s, were being taken from the land and put in prison camps. The total heart-beating chicken flesh in those places now exceeds the mass of birds in the sky.

I am frequently asked what kind of a world I want and am fighting for. I want a world where people cherish the lives that we share and where ethics and intelligence come together to make the best life possible for every bird, every being in every habitat on Earth. I want a world where the crow of a rooster, the cluck of a hen, the cheeping of chicks, and the whole joyous commotion of birds bounce off the branches, echo through the earth, and fill the sky with heart and voice. I want—and I work for—a world where all is well because the avian soul is satisfied and because, as Emily Dickinson wrote:

> "Hope" is the thing with feathers—
> That perches in the soul—
> And sings the tune without the words—
> And never stops—at all.[37]

The greatest challenge for me as an activist is knowing what chickens and other birds are going through everywhere on Earth all the time. The big categories are extinction, incarceration, and endless proliferation of avian beings in industrial incarceration. It isn't only the birds, of course; it's the whole scene, the moral injury we inflict on our fellow creatures of other species with almost no—if any—remorse or restitution.

The easiest part of my work is being with the birds in our sanctuary: To be in their company, to share the day with them, to be able to help them and experience their enthusiasm bring joy. As when Rowdy the rooster looks me in the eye and then crows his heart out in what I like to think of as a proclamation of our kindred spirits and primal accord.

MARY FINELLI

Founder and President, Fish Feel

Mary Finelli is the founder and president of Fish Feel, the first organization focused on promoting the recognition of fishes as sentient beings deserving of respect and compassion. Mary also chairs the Save the Rays Coalition. She has a BS in animal science and has been active in animal rights advocacy since the mid-1980s. Mary has worked with various animal protection organizations, primarily focusing on farmed animals. She produced *Farmed Animal Watch*, a weekly online news digest sponsored by numerous animal protection organizations, and co-wrote a chapter of *In Defense of Animals: The Second Wave*.

SWIMMING AGAINST IGNORANCE AND CRUELTY

"She won't eat anything."

"Try tuna."

My mother's advice to my grandmother worked. Aside from milk, it was the only thing my fifteen-month-old self would consume until my mother returned home from the hospital after having given birth to my sister Darlene. All the while I was growing up, seafood was my favorite food: tuna salad, fish sticks, shrimp, lobster, clam chowder, cream of oyster soup. I loved it all. As with so many people who become vegetarian, aquatic animals were the last animals I stopped eating. If only I'd known then what I know now!

Eating aquatic animals causes the most animal suffering. Like so many other people, I didn't think of them in the same way I thought of mammals or birds. Even though I had been an extremely empathic child and had truly loved the few companion goldfishes we'd had, and while I came to realize that eating other animals was morally wrong, the wrongness of eating fish just didn't register. In fact, I turned without compunction to eating more fishes after quitting eating other animals.

What the hell was wrong with me? The same problem that afflicts so many other people: cultural ignorance and desensitization. Why feel bad for tunas when Charlie the Tuna was so disappointed to not have been caught by StarKist fishermen? After all, vegetarians eat fish, don't they? And isn't fishing a wholesome, peaceful pastime? Fishes don't even feel pain, do they? Society is bad enough when it comes to our perception of other animals, but it is absolutely appalling in regard to consideration of fishes.

While it should be plainly apparent to any sensible person that fishes can indeed suffer pain, there are even some scientists who continue to dispute that they do. The plethora of compelling scientific evidence should dispel any doubts that fishes are sentient, but there is great incentive for the public to believe that they aren't: the appetite for fish flesh and the popularity of fish oil, the multi-billion-dollar fishing and fish-farming industries, the heavy reliance on the use of fishes for experimental research, the popularity of "recreational" fishing and the immense amount of money made catering to those who participate in it, the interest in keeping fishes captive for entertainment and the lucrative industries that capture or breed them for it, and so on.

However, fish sentience is growing increasingly difficult to dispute, with ever-accumulating scientific evidence and the growing public realization that fishes do indeed suffer fear and pain and are admirable beings who deserve respect, compassion, and moral consideration. As ethologist Jonathan Balcombe, author of the very informative book *What a Fish Knows*, explains: "fish have personalities, they plan, recognize, remember, court, parent, innovate, manipulate, collaborate, communicate with gestures, keep accounts, deduce, deceive, show virtue, form attachments, have traditions, fall for optical illusions, get depressed, use tools, learn by observation, and form mental maps."[38]

Entities ranging from the Smithsonian Institution to the American Veterinary Medical Association have recognized that fishes can experience pain. They are keenly sensitive animals, trillions of whom are made to suffer intensely by the fishing industry every year. Caught on hooks or in massive nets, they can be left hanging in agony for days, and common slaughter methods can actually prolong their suffering.

These indiscriminate fishing methods also catch many millions of birds, dolphins, seals, turtles, and whales each year, many of whom are thrown back dead or dying. Trawling, whereby heavy nets are dragged along the ocean floor, also catch indiscriminately while destroying fragile coral reefs and other habitats. In addition, animals who compete with humans for fish are intentionally killed. Much of this carnage is made possible with heavy government subsidies. As if this weren't bad enough, human slavery is rampant in the fishing industry, much of whose catch is consumed in the US and Europe.

Many—if not most—of the fishes who are caught are used as feed for farmed fishes (and farmed crabs, chickens, minks, pigs, and shrimps), so fishing props up those cruel industries, too. Fish farming tends to be grossly inefficient, with more fishes used as feed than produced. It is also egregiously inhumane. The fishes are kept captive in crowded pens that are polluted with feces and decomposing feed. Diseases can quickly spread through the pens, so antibiotics and other chemicals are heavily used. The captive fishes are often heavily infested with parasitic sea lice, and procedures to get rid of them can be lethal to the fishes. Ocean-based fish farms pollute the surrounding water, and lice and disease can be transmitted through the caging to wild fishes. As with wild-caught fishes, slaughter methods for farmed fishes are brutal and can prolong their suffering.

Despite the many health hazards that fish consumption presents (e.g., mercury, dioxins, PCBs, parasites, microplastics, cholesterol, saturated fat), the government and even the medical community continue to promote it. Many people who give up "red meat" switch to eating more birds and fishes, greatly increasing the number of animals they cause to be killed. Fish oil is similarly problematic. Despite being long touted as beneficial for an array of ailments, fish oil is continually found not only to fail to help but to be a potential health hazard. In addition to being potentially contaminated, it can quickly become rancid, which may increase the risk of inflammation, atherosclerosis, organ damage, and cancer.

We started Fish Feel because there was such a gaping lack of concern for fishes, even within the animal protection community. Fortunately, the past few years have seen growing appreciation of them and attention to their plight. "Friends not food" (from the fish-friendly movie *Finding Nemo*) has become a popular slogan. The 2017 book *What a Fish Knows* is a bestseller that has been translated into fifteen languages. Vegan seafood recipes and products are quickly growing in diversity and popularity. Advocacy and activism for fishes are also increasing, with more animal protection organizations beginning to campaign for them. Interest in fish issues seems similar now to what interest in chicken issues was like about twenty years ago. Interest in welfare improvements for farmed fishes, in particular, is growing globally.

With little to no legal protection, fishes desperately need all of the help they can get. However, decades of efforts to improve conditions for other farmed animals have proven woefully disappointing, and what little legal protection they do have tends to give the public false assurance that they are treated humanely. Welfare certification systems are similarly misleading, and certification programs for fishes rarely even include welfare factors. The public needs to realize that there is no genuinely humane way to fish, or to raise and slaughter animals; this needs to be made clear to people.

What really is needed is genuine respect for fishes and other animals—our fellow sentient beings. As long as it is considered socially acceptable to intentionally torture and kill animals for fun (so-called "recreational" fishing), society will remain far from that goal. It is especially alarming that industry, government, and charities are making such a big push to get children, women, and disabled people to take up fishing. It is antithetical to veganism.

It's truly an atrocity that nonhuman animals continue to be treated so horrifically in this day and age. I think of how obtuse I was toward fishes, and it helps temper my aggravation with nonvegans. Public perception of nonhuman animals is improving though, and there are fewer and fewer excuses for such ignorance. As for apathy, it is inexcusable.

I still enjoy seafood, but now I choose from many delicious vegan versions. All of the nutrients we need in order to thrive can be obtained more healthfully, humanely, and environmentally responsibly from plant sources, and there are marvelous vegan versions of virtually every type of food imaginable.

PETE AND KIT JAGODA

Co-founders, River's Wish Animal Sanctuary

Pete and Kit Jagoda co-founded and operate River's Wish Animal Sanctuary in Spokane, Washington. Their rescue work began in 1994 and they incorporated as a 501c3 in 2005. They care for approximately 140 farmed animals on their sixty-five-acre sanctuary with a team of extraordinary volunteers and supporters. As artists and teachers, they integrate art with their Sanctuary Based Education Programs. Pete has an MFA in sculpture and teaches jewelry at Spokane Falls Community College. He creates reliquaries and sculptures at the sanctuary. Kit is in her thirty-third year of teaching art full-time in public schools. She holds a Masters in Humane Education from the Institute for Humane Education and Valparaiso University. The Jagodas advocate vegan living for ethical reasons.

SANCTUARY: THIS IS WHAT MATTERS

In the spring of 1994, we responded to an ad in the newspaper seeking foster homes for shelter dogs and cats. Within a week of our answering the ad, our perspective was beginning to shift dramatically. Seeing the high numbers of homeless dogs and cats, many of whom would be euthanized, was shocking. We wondered why this was not common knowledge. Where was the outrage against society's failing these beloved companions?

This jolt of reality was the gateway to our growing awareness of the plight of *all* animals. From dogs and cats to the "pet" industry, farmed animals, wildlife, and sea life, the truth was and continues to be horrific and undeniable.

We had a very strong bond with our dog River, whom Kit adopted in 1986. He was a family member, and we knew him as an individual.

Our experience getting into the rescue world introduced us to so many individuals and their needs, which fostered deeper compassion and empathy. This empathy grew to extend beyond the boundaries of individuals we had met, to the billions who are harmed by humans every year. This took us beyond ourselves and into a life we had never imagined. A life we would never change.

Rescue and rehabilitation enveloped us and before long, we were building shelters and fences, and running electrical and water lines— all to accommodate animals in need. Our sixty-five-acre home would become a place of peace for those seeking sanctuary. We felt driven to do what we could to make a difference for at least a few.

We named our all-volunteer organization River's Wish Animal Sanctuary after our beloved golden dog; it would be a place where others could find peace and be free from harm. Recently, a dear friend passed, and in honor of her, we are integrating "Diana's Dream" into our Sanctuary Based Education Program. Her dream was that everyone would see each animal as an individual and respect their right to live and be loved.

Over the years, we have rescued dogs from spending their entire lives on chains; safely captured and cared for warrens of domestic feral rabbits; saved horses, goats, sheep, pigs, birds, and bovines from slaughter; and given hope to countless individuals whose lives were in peril. However, for all that we have been able to provide for them, they have given back so much more, and in this we all seem to find sanctuary.

These are just the stories of a few of the remarkable individuals whom we have been fortunate to call friends:

Paloma

In 2005, we were able to save a former PMU (Pregnant Mare Urine, a.k.a. Premarin) Percheron from slaughter. When she arrived at the sanctuary, she was thin, muddy, and extremely fearful. She had no reason to trust humans. Humans had mistreated her in the exploitive PMU industry, and she was going to be shipped to slaughter. We named her Paloma (the Spanish word for "dove"), for despite all of her mistrust, she carried a gentle essence about her. After a short time of being with us, Paloma had a severe episode of colic. We drove her seventy miles south to the

Washington State University veterinary hospital, where she underwent surgery to remove twelve feet of intestine that had lodged in a hole in her diaphragm. The veterinarian said it was caused by a congenital condition, but she felt positive that Paloma could lead a long and healthy life.

Paloma remained at WSU for the following two months. Over the course of this time, she basically "owned" the veterinary students who were responsible for taking her for walks, cleaning her stall, and keeping a watchful eye on her. During this time, Paloma's confidence and trust grew. She learned that humans could also be kind and loving. She taught us the importance of never giving up and not betraying trust. Paloma is now one of our friendliest equines. She follows people, loves attention, and even joins our Art and Animal Workshops. We refer to her as "your basic two-thousand-pound puppy dog." Paloma embodies the very essence of learning to trust after a lifetime of betrayal.

Rudy

Rudy was a young Jersey steer when he was brought to us by the local animal protection agency after being seized in a cruelty case. Rudy was our introduction to bovines, and it didn't take long for us to realize he needed a companion. Dr. Scott, one of our veterinarians, offered to bring his elderly cow Yula to live with Rudy. Yula taught Rudy all things bovine. He became calmer in her presence and seemed to respect her matriarchal position. When Yula passed, we were all very sad, but Rudy's grief was palpable. He stood steadfast by her body as Pete prepared her grave. When Pete gently lowered Yula into the grave, Rudy followed her down the slope. He stood beside her, bellowing the most mournful sound. Pete stepped down from the tractor and joined Rudy. They mourned Yula together. Over the following weeks, Rudy was a lone silhouette when there had formerly been two. He was grieving and we felt so helpless.

During this time, our friend Sue, founder of New Dawn Montana Farm Sanctuary, passed from a long battle with cancer. We promised to care for her two steers, Henry and Bergh. The boys made the trip from Montana to Spokane on November 22, 2014. Rudy welcomed them with a dance of jumps and leaps as he joyfully entered their space. It was deeply moving to experience Rudy's grieving process, and it was hopeful to witness how his new companions brought light back into his life. This sanctuary life is profoundly spiritual.

During sanctuary visits, children have asked, "Do animals have emotions?" Pete would revisit the story of Rudy and Yula, shedding light on the deeply emotional lives of the animals. Each time he retells this story, his eyes well with tears. Being witness to such an array of emotions is a gift we are grateful for. In fact, just as much as Rudy was joyful when meeting Henry and Bergh, he has shown emotion toward music. During our annual Art for the Animals benefit auction each summer, Rudy leans over the fence and is seemingly soothed. Of the different varieties of music, it is the blues that draws him closer. Rudy loves the blues.

Delilah

Delilah was a queen, and the first pig we brought to the sanctuary. Her previous life was unknown as she was a stray. Delilah was intelligent, curious, and regal, and would welcome the other pigs as they arrived at the sanctuary. She loved mud baths, belly scratches, and ear rubs. She loved Rudy when he first arrived, and she loved all her little pig companions who came to rest under her matriarchy. Alice, Dwin, Ennis, Lil Pig, and Miss Piggy held Delilah in the highest regard.

When the time came and we had to help Delilah leave her tired old body behind, her family stayed near. They surrounded her. It was their turn to protect the one who had always kept them safe. Following the euthanasia, her family continued to remain by her side. They covered her body with the surrounding hay and lay with her throughout the remainder of the night.

Animals share their deep emotions with one another, and if one is fortunate to witness even a bit of this, one has received a great gift. We believe it is our duty to share this story with our fellow humans to give a glimpse into another individual's life. This is the least we can do for our nonhuman friends.

Life at a Sanctuary

Sanctuary life is not easy. It is all-consuming. It takes its toll physically, mentally, and emotionally. It is the fact that sanctuary matters so much to so many that keeps us on this path. This path involves endless fundraising throughout the year and being aware of the limits of our resources, whether human, financial, or environmental. It requires establishing boundaries and identifying our own emotions, yet maintaining flexibility in order to best meet the needs of the animals. It requires that we let go of what we thought our life was going to be, let go of ideas of vacations and of boredom. It means holding on to hope and possibilities while healing broken hearts. It is a never-ending learning process.

People think they would like to start a sanctuary, and more sanctuaries are surely needed, but keep in mind that this is a 24/7 commitment: cleaning, feeding, medicating, fixing, mending, going to the vet, fundraising, supporting volunteers, worrying, continuing to stick with it, staying with the residents, being with them when they pass no matter how much it hurts, and not giving up. It will become your way of life. *Your life.* It will define what you do and when you do it. It will change you. Be ready to be changed in ways that you never imagined. You can never unsee what you'll have seen. You will be in the trenches; you will trudge through the mud, slide on the ice while trying not to break through it, and watch and prepare for any storms and fires that may come. And in the midst of it all, you seek moments to hold a precious animal whose life you were able to impact and who definitely impacted yours.

We initially entered this work to help nonhuman animals, and it organically grew into a way of living, an example and manifest presence of "This Is What Matters." It is a continual drive to do all we can within our power to make a difference in the lives of the individuals in our care and of those we meet along the way. We have an amazing group of dedicated volunteers and supporters who make all of this possible. Our long-range plans are for River's Wish to continue into the future beyond us, providing a space of peace, refuge, and education.

Art and Education

As visual artists and art teachers, we know that education is key to raising awareness, hearts and minds, and empathy. We have developed a Sanctuary Based Education Program that includes Art and Animal

Workshops, Garden to Table Workshops, and Compassionate Living Workshops. We hold sanctuary visits, field trips, and events from spring through fall. We value the relationship between art, education, advocacy, rescue, and sanctuary—five key elements in the work we do at River's Wish, which are also central to our personal lives. To be able to connect these elements and share them with others through sanctuary-based education is an opportunity to impact change.

When visitors meet the residents and hear their stories, we hope this opens hearts and minds to the plight of animals directly affected by human action. So many individuals come to the sanctuary from dire situations or have been removed from the animal agriculture industry. Through developing and fostering genuine empathy for these individuals, we hope this sentiment will also extend toward the billions of other nonhuman animals who are harmed every year, other humans, and the environment.

Through our sanctuary-based education, we aim to replace the abstract notion of a nonhuman species, of a "food animal" with a connection to an individual. We utilize art to communicate our recognition that social justice issues are at the center of how animals are regarded. Visual art is capable of speaking volumes about social justice themes in ways that may not be articulated through words.

The experience of sharing our lives with the sanctuary residents gives us a unique opportunity to practice critical thinking and problem solving from a both practical and theoretical point of view. Our knowledge grows from experience coupled with ethics. And always central to our lives is gratitude. We are grateful to provide a space for individuals to find peace. We are grateful for the humans who volunteer and visit, and for those we are able to help. We are grateful for the support we receive and for our connections with the growing compassion for nonhuman animals.

There is grief and there is joy in all of this—whether it be grief from losing a precious resident, from the inability to help someone in need, or joy for those lives we can touch and impact. We all become a nurturing part of each other's lives here. At our sanctuary, this is so much of what really matters.

INGRID NEWKIRK

President and Founder, People for the Ethical Treatment of Animals (PETA)

Ingrid Newkirk is the founder and president of People for the Ethical Treatment of Animals (PETA), the largest animal rights organization in the world with more than 6.5 million members and supporters worldwide. She is the author of more than a dozen books that have been translated into several languages, her latest being *Animalkind: Remarkable Discoveries about Animals and Revolutionary New Ways to Show Them Compassion.*

A BIRTHDAY SURPRISE

We were at the fanciest restaurant that served lobster in the Philadelphia area, and we had driven hours to get there. It was my birthday, and I can't remember now if I was turning twenty or somewhere around there. The place was gorgeous—that I do remember—and the evening was perfect. White wine, freshly baked bread, candles, white linen, soft music, and the man I loved beside me. We ordered the lobster.

The next thing I recall is the waiter arriving with a silver salver, on which there were three lobsters to choose from. They waved their antennae in our direction, but I thought nothing of it. I didn't know then that lobsters flirt, hold hands to guide each other across the ocean floor, and live to be decades old. I also didn't know what my next words would mean to the one I gestured toward as I said, in answer to the question, "Broiled or boiled?": "Broiled, please."

The lobsters were taken away, and we returned to our happy talk about our new little house in the Maryland countryside, our dog, and our plans. Our meal arrived a little later. The lobster meat was fluffed up in the middle and the claws were huge and bursting with cooked, pinkish-red flesh. I squeezed lemon onto the lump on my fork and popped it into my mouth.

What happened next was totally unexpected. I burst into tears.

The subconscious is an interesting thing. It takes on board bits of information, and while you are otherwise occupied, it sets out to process them, even concluding things from them without your having any idea this is going on. In this case, my subconscious had apparently realized that the lobsters, not having the power of speech at their disposal, had attempted to communicate in the only manner they could—by waving their antennae at us. Somewhere in the recesses of my mind, there had taken place a realization that this was a cry for help. Just as a dog who cannot ask to be let out may scratch at the door or bring you a leash, the lobsters seemed to have been signaling their panic, their fear, their desire to be returned to their ocean home.

What I did know was that when I lifted my fork and placed the warm lump of lobster in my mouth, that subconscious thought worked its way forward. It was as if someone had upturned the wine bucket and poured the ice over my head. I suddenly understood that I had glibly taken another living being's life and was now eating the dead body to celebrate my own life.

It was only much later that I learned that when you ask that a live lobster be broiled, the lobster is split down the back with a sharp knife, pats of butter are inserted into the wound, salt and pepper are sprinkled on top, and the animal is then slid under the red-hot grill.

That gap in my knowledge notwithstanding, I knew from that moment on that there would be no more cracking open of steamed crabs, no more shrimp cocktails, no more lobster salad. I couldn't bring back the lobster I had just killed, but I could be sure that I would never kill another lobster—or any other animal—because I could now relate to who was on my plate.

Fifty years on, there are innumerable nonviolently produced "taste-alikes"—mock lobster, crab, and shrimp among them. Our Japanese restaurant up the street serves them all. I don't need them, but if I fancy them, they are there.

I am glad we have a subconscious and the "mirror neurons" that allow us to put ourselves in the place of even the "oddest," most alien beings, who seem the furthest removed from us. Practicing empathy, understanding, and respect can only be a good thing after all.

RAE SIKORA

International Speaker, Educator, Writer

Rae Sikora has been a spokesperson for other species and the environment for over forty years. Her interactive critical-thinking trainings and talks have been presented around the globe. Rae is the co-founder of The Institute for Humane Education, VegFund, Santa Fe Vegan, and Plant Peace Daily. She and her partner Jim "JC" Corcoran co-founded Root 66 Vegan Café and Catering. They live in Santa Fe, New Mexico, with their pack of rescue dogs.

THERE IS NO OTHER

How many of you have experienced the frustration of being seen as part of some group rather than as an individual? Personally, I don't want to be seen as just a woman or just an old person or just an American or just a white person. There is something in humans that makes it difficult for us not to judge an individual based on their group. The judgment is often based on a meaningless physical characteristic or a cultural difference. Within our own species, it is challenging for us not to judge another based on how they look, their language, their sexual orientation, their gender, their education level, etc. Also, if we do not share the same language and culture, it is difficult for us to understand another human. We do not know if the other person is funny, intelligent, or what we have in common with them because we are so strongly oriented to verbal connections.

Years ago, I experienced a lesson in this. It was one of my first wake-up calls to my own judgmental attitudes. I was working at a peace camp in Costa Rica. We were a large group of volunteers from all over the world working on getting the camp built and ready to open. I was in charge of three of the smaller groups. I would buzz around on a bicycle and give directions to the three groups. One of the groups was nine women from an indigenous tribe who were there volunteering, and it was the first time they had ventured out of their small village. Their job was to paint the entrance sign for the camp. I left them with yellow paint, brushes, and ladders. Our common language was Spanish, but none of us was fluent. I asked them to paint the carved letters on the giant brown sign yellow. Then I got on the bike to check on another group. When I got back to the women, they were all laughing, covered in splattered yellow paint. The sign and the ground under it were a mess of yellow drips and puddles. I asked them to show me what had happened, and one of them demonstrated how they had been dipping the brushes into the cans and throwing paint onto the sign. What I learned was that they had never seen a paintbrush or painted and didn't know the step of dragging the brush along the edge of the can to get the excess paint off. I thought, *This is going to be a long couple of weeks. These women don't have many skills.* The next day, the caretaker brought a truckload of machetes to me and these same women and told us to clear an area for a cabin. The women each grabbed a machete and went to the rocks nearby and started sharpening them on the rocks. I stood there with my machete, clueless about how to sharpen it. When they asked me what was wrong, I told them I had never sharpened a machete before. They all looked at each other and I can almost guarantee they were thinking, *This is going to be a long couple of weeks. This woman doesn't know much.*

This taught me an important lesson. We learn the skills necessary to survive in our own culture and our own circumstances. Intelligence and skills are not one-size-fits-all. It also made me think about how easy it is to misunderstand and judge someone of our own species. And that led me to a better understanding of how easy it is to misjudge another species. We do not share other animals' cultures and languages. As with other humans, unless we spend a lot of time with an individual of any other species, it is easy to see them as simply a member of their group. I have seen people who met a pig or a cow or a chicken for the first time have that experience completely change their idea about that group. Beyond rescuing nonhuman individuals and giving them a good life, this is one of the great benefits of animal sanctuaries. Most people are forever changed when they connect one-on-one with farmed animals, monkeys, chimpanzees, elephants, and others at a sanctuary.

Most of the injustices in the world stem from the inability to see a thinking, feeling individual in another living being. Slavery, abuse, and murder of innocent beings are not limited to our own species. It is still challenging for humans to care about all humans, so it is not surprising that we are limited in our ability to care about all species. Why can many humans care so deeply about one species and not care about another? There are people who love dogs or cats but feel nothing when it comes to the animals they choose to eat or wear. There are hunters who love their dogs but easily shoot those of other species. Many people are excited to eat their holiday ham or turkey but would be horrified if a dog or cat were roasted and served. The difference with the dog or cat is that we know individuals of those species. We have welcomed them into our homes. We have called them "family."

My dear friends from Kenya used to talk about how LGBT people were the "sick ones in the human species" and should either be killed or be put on a separate island so they wouldn't weaken our species. After months of their being with all my friends, I asked them who was their favorite. They all said Sarah. I asked them, "Why Sarah?" They replied that Sarah was the kindest, funniest, smartest, and most beautiful. When I told them that Sarah was a lesbian (I had asked Sarah's permission to tell them), they laughed. When they saw me not laughing, they sat in shock. "Sarah can't be a lesbian—you are joking, right? We love her. It is impossible she is a lesbian." In the months and years to come, this Kenyan family became the most outspoken advocates for LGBT rights in the Kenyan expat community. Knowing and caring about one individual had opened their hearts to the entire LGBT community.

Much of our work on Earth is to find compassion for those who are different from us. The definition of *compassion* in Merriam-Webster Dictionary is: "sympathetic consciousness of others' distress together with a desire to alleviate it."

Who is included in our circle of caring and compassion is often determined by whether they are familiar to us and whether we have connected with them in some way. If we let go of fear and take the time to connect with other living beings, even the most unfamiliar, we would never see their groups in the same way again.

Which groups of humans and which species do you still have strong judgments of? Whom do you see as different from you and less deserving of compassion? You can make this your challenge: Find someone in that group and connect with them. Get to know them as an individual. Whether it is the homeless person asking for money on the street corner or the chicken living in a sanctuary near you, take the time to find out who they really are. You will be forever changed.

JESSE TANDLER

Educational Program Director, Factory Farming
Awareness Coalition (FFAC)

A writer, academic, and educator for over a decade and a half, Jesse Tandler began teaching high school students about the ethics of our food culture in 2008. During his PhD work, he continued to include our treatment of animals on the syllabi of his undergraduate classes at the City University of New York, where for five years he taught philosophy, literature, writing, and rhetoric. In 2017, he moved to Los Angeles to apply his years of research and educational experience in the nonprofit sphere. He also teaches food politics at UCLA.

WHAT KIND OF PERSON AM I?

In 2013, two of my oldest and closest friends visited me in New York. As we sat in a random Midtown diner, the topic of dog abuse came up. One of my friends began to vent about people who mistreat their dogs. "It makes me sick," he said. "Those people should be shot." When I ventured that we treat cows, pigs, and other farmed animals the same—even worse—he said quietly and with finality, "That's different."

Whatever I feel now notwithstanding, for much of my life I would have adamantly agreed with him and spun various rationales for the completely normal behavior of treating one animal with love and another as a thing to turn into a meal. I saw nothing wrong with this. My parents and grandparents—all moral and caring people—ate other animals, as did the majority of my friends. I say "other" because we, of course, are also animals. The whole process seemed in sync with nature. I remember saying on more than one occasion that animals tasted like I was supposed to eat them. How else could I explain the sensation of raw tuna dissolving deliciously between my teeth and upper palate? Or the visceral satisfaction from delicately marinated *kalbi* tearing cleanly from a rib bone?

The pleasure confirmed the obvious choice to continue enjoying what I'd always enjoyed, what my parents and grandparents had taught me to enjoy. Plus, beyond the pleasure of the meal, there were the loving associations. What would Thanksgiving be without the traditional turkey and my Uncle Sandy's stuffing? What would *dim sum* be without my high school friends divvying up little baskets of *shumai*?

Not only did I eat other animals, but I was suspicious of people who didn't. This attitude was no secret to my friends. An ex-girlfriend has often reminded me of something I said on our first date. We'd met for Ethiopian food. One of the globs on our shared plate consisted of a baby sheep ground to bits and simmered in a spicy sauce. Scooping some into my mouth, I said I'd never be with a vegetarian. Giving up one of life's most consistent pleasures seemed unimaginable, even wrong.

Slowly, however, several incidents forced my imagination into the spaces my food had inhabited. One evening, my ex and I were cuddling on the couch, watching a documentary. The film, though falling far short of advocating vegetarianism, showed footage—even if rather tame—of cows in factory farms. The cows stood literally knee-deep in ponds of their own waste. They looked uncomfortable wading through it. Flies swarmed the dried cakes of excrement on their flanks and backs. My ex said, "We probably shouldn't eat them." I couldn't bring myself to disagree. The conditions were awful. Even if I enjoyed eating cows, this wasn't okay. And the pigs had it worse. Though neither of us stopped eating these creatures, my food, once just a slab on a plate, began to take on the form of an animal with a history—a life of walking around in fear, pain, and excrement, ending finally with a bolt through the brain or a blade to the throat. In me, at least, there surfaced a consciousness—or conscience—in the form of an openness to alternatives.

Probably because my desires were open to a change of perspective, I allowed myself to seek out information. Soon, I stopped buying factory-farmed animal flesh. I didn't want to support the demand for it and convinced myself that grass-fed cows were the moral option. They got to roam around and have a decent life, right? Everyone dies at some point anyway, so if they lived happy lives and were killed "humanely," what objection could there be?

With my new restriction, sometimes I'd eat an animal from the sea or consume flesh at restaurants that claimed to source from "ethical" farms rather than some version of a concentration camp. The reduction in meat improved my physical wellbeing. Constipation had almost ceased to be a problem. Morally, too, I felt I could applaud myself for contributing significantly less destruction to the planet and to our water supply. My decisions felt good—aside from when I once had a bite of my omnivorous friend Paul's leftovers and was met with accusations of inconsistency.

"It's a sentient being," he said.

"It's dead," I replied. "I didn't order it. I'm not increasing any demand for suffering, merely not letting it go to waste. Many Buddhists do the same."

"Jess, you can't eat any sentient beings if you believe it's wrong to harm them. Period." His charges of inconsistency annoyed me. I knew I felt a deep affection for animals, and I believed it was wrong to make them suffer unnecessarily. But I was loath to give up eating them and needed a solid justification to absolve my having them murdered for my pleasure. Someone smarter than me must have come up with an argument I wasn't aware of, so as I often do, I turned to books. Starting with the ancients and moving up to the present, I searched for logic to validate my hope. But the more I read, the more I had to admit that Paul had a point. Not only is eating animals unnecessary for survival, but it's even unhealthy according to the best science. Further, if I believed it wrong to murder a human, then the fundamental arguments for such a belief should also apply to other social, sentient individuals. The only reason I might value a human animal's life over another animal's life is because I am a human animal and can understand the loss better. It's not because a human's life is in any way intrinsically more valuable to the human than a cow's life is to the cow. Animals demonstrate an unequivocal will to live, as I learned when I tried to coax a cat into a mobile carrier.

I had to conclude that remaining a meat eater in any capacity or exploiting female animals in painful ways for their milk and eggs made sense only by a selfish calculus predicated on my palatal pleasure and convenience.

But there was something else I realized.

In the course of my conversations with friends and family, at the point where they couldn't deny the logic, they'd usually fall back on, "Animals are just different." Or: "I don't really care about animals. I just can't. They're not people."

Each time, I felt frustrated. Yes, a human isn't a cow. A cow isn't a dog. A dog isn't a pig. So what? What's the essential difference that insists we treat humans with dignity, as ends in themselves, but treat other animals as means to our ends?

Because of where I am in history, because of the activism of my grandparents and people like them, because of the anti-Semitism (albeit mild) I've experienced, because of the racism I've witnessed toward my friends, I've grown up viewing race as the result of a tribalistic hierarchy that apportions value based on skin-deep features. Race imagines a division between "us" and "them." But what's really the difference? By all important measures, aren't "they" "us" as much as *we* are? What makes the dissolution of racial, sexual, or otherwise arbitrary boundaries vital is our knowledge that others have bodies that feel pain and pleasure as ours do, have families and loved ones as we do—loved ones who, like us, grieve loss. According to this logic, the classification of "species" is an equally vicious boundary and a prejudice that, like race, excuses our desire to harvest amusement and utility from others' bodies.

If you've lived with a nonhuman animal, you know that nonhuman animals' bodies are sensitive, often more sensitive than our own, and that their emotions are intense and meaningful to them. My dog Sabbath certainly got more excited about his next meal or walk than does any human I know. And had I hung him upside down and knifed his throat, the pain and confusion in his brown eyes would have been as real as my mother's, my father's, my sister's, or my own.

With this realization, I was unable to continue seeing other animals as "them." To justify eating other animals, I had to commodify their bodies and judge their lives and emotions as less important than the brief pleasure from chewing their flesh. I had to generally objectify them as some*things*—rather than some*ones*—that I could chop to pieces, dip in a sauce, and sauté with onions, garlic, and tomatoes, while oiling the pan to keep their muscles from sticking to the burning metal. As a result, a steak or a pork chop was no longer food but the history and horrific abbreviation of a life. I couldn't unsee it. Every steak was *Sabbath* on the plate. All ribs were *Sabbath's* ribs. And it went a step further. That was *me* on the plate. Those were *my* ribs.

The Jewish Nobel laureate Isaac Bashevis Singer wrote: "In their behavior toward creatures, all men are Nazis. The smugness with which man can do with other species as he pleases exemplifies the most extreme racist theories, the principle that might is right."[39] These days, I try not to be so certain of my views. However, if I've come to any certainty about how to treat others, it's that I'd rather act with love than with selfishness, and not allow my power over them to convince me of my right to do them harm. Instead of echoing the Nazi, I'd rather follow the example of the Buddha, who noted: "All beings tremble before violence. All love life. All fear death. See yourself in others. Then whom can you hurt?"[40]

A couple of friends have said that my position is extreme. But is it really extreme to act with the intentions of love, kindness, and empathy? I'm happy to be questioning the privilege I have as a male, as a heterosexual, as a light-skinned person, as a human. It allows me to recognize the discrimination inherent in accepting as a matter of course the domination of men over women, heterosexuals over nonheterosexuals, whites over nonwhites, and finally, human animals over nonhuman animals—i.e., human individuals over other *individuals.*

I understand some people feel judged by my position. But the irony of my past self is not lost on my current self. While it upsets me that people, particularly those I care about, go on treating other animals as unfeeling objects, claiming the objectification and murder of the animals are a matter of "personal choice," the irony keeps me from standing in judgment. How could I be judgmental when for about three decades I regularly dismissed other animals' lives as less important than the taste of their dismembered bodies? I also fully understand the fear of missing out on certain comfort foods, or of being perceived as different or weird. Those fears were mine, too. Even once I stopped eating other animals' bodies, I still feared giving up milk and eggs, a fear I shed a year or so later. The fears, in the end, were unwarranted. I am healthier, eat delicious food, and have concluded that not only can I live agreeably without exploiting other animals, but I can live better.

When confronted with any moral decision, I've learned to ask myself, "What kind of human do I want to be?" In response, I do my best to be the kind of human who is honest and generous toward my tribe and others, toward children of humans and children of other animals. Because I no longer can imagine any intrinsic difference between murdering a dog and murdering a pig or a fish or a human, I choose to be the kind of person who eats plants—nutritious, bloodless plants. No other decision in my life has given me such a sense of strength or harmony.

So when I ask, "What kind of person am I?" I know that with every decision I make, with every instance I choose kindness over selfishness, empathy over fear, vegetables over pig, I'm finding an answer to that question.

SECTION TWO
Around the Globe

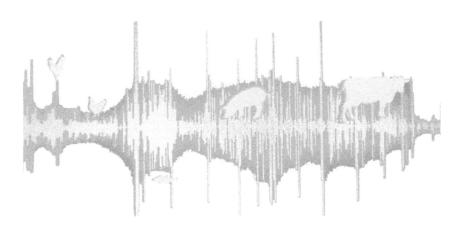

ELIN GUNDERSEN

Vegan Grassroots Organizer

Elin Gundersen is a creative concept developer, writer, and coach. Her passion is to spread awareness about the need for a simpler, more sustainable lifestyle. In 2016, she opened vegan café Greenseed with André Gundersen, and in 2017, they created a vegan festival, Green Food Fest. In 2020, along with Kristine Rykkelid and Erik Musum, they founded a development company for sustainable vegan concepts, Greenseed Norge AS. Building concepts, bridgework, and collaboration for improving the world, they enable and inspire people to go vegan. They invite co-creators to contribute to all their platforms, including vegan lifestyle blog *Make a Momentum*. They will make history when they open LOCO, Norway's first full-range vegan grocery store chain.

UNDERSTANDING THE POWER OF COMPASSION

Fighting for Peace

I was adopted at thirteen months old and brought up in a Seventh-Day Adventist household. As with veganism, I loved how religious texts spoke highly of love, compassion, and kindness. But in reality, I witnessed how interpretations of the words were also used to justify judgment, hate, and violence. This hypocrisy didn't fare well with me; nevertheless, I myself was also guilty. Growing up, I just wanted everyone to get along, to be fine and happy. Some people seemed unfazed when witnessing cruelty, but I could feel the pain of every living organism through my bones, as if it were my own. Everywhere I turned, hearts were broken, wounds were opened, and I wondered why I was placed here, if only to suffer. I couldn't handle the pain, so I made up strategies to avoid it or try to stop it. I worked hard every day to encourage common understandings to prevent conflict.

My constantly rejected peacemaking efforts made me adopt the belief that I wasn't good enough. I couldn't separate myself from what I perceived to be my failed accomplishments—not being able to make everything right or to let go if something was wrong. It led me to believe that I wasn't deserving of love, kindness, or happiness. In my late twenties, I began to grasp that my self-proclaimed responsibility to single-handedly save the world was—well—crazy. I also realized that my drive to fix things had worked as a distraction from addressing my own problems.

Everyone is doing the best they can with what they have and what they know at any one time. If we could do better, we would. Holding on to regrets and judging ourselves for not being unrealistically successful aren't serving anyone.

We need to be able to forgive ourselves and accept that it's okay not to be perfect. Until we can do that, we'll hold ourselves captive in an imaginary prison of self-inflicted suffering based on our own negative distortions—inhibited from taking charge of our lives.

Connecting the Dots

We can't outrun unpleasantness; it will always catch up with us. If we can accept that and stop interpreting it as a personal punishment or a sign of weakness, we can use it as never-ending motivation to fuel necessary change. We can't change our circumstances instantly, but we can take action, create, interact, and respond to ourselves and others through the lens of kindness.

If I've learned anything in this life, it's that living your life as a victim is a choice. The only person who can hold yourself back is you! Essentially, *you* are the person behind all of your problems. We can wire our brains to find evidence to support our negative illusions about what we are capable of, or we can accept the unpleasantness and employ it to forge new paths.

In 2016, I went on a program called Vegan Reset to help stabilize my mood and energy levels and to take better care of my mental health.

Suddenly, everything clicked into place. I discovered how aligning my actions with my core values and sense of compassion made me feel so much better about myself. Embracing a lifestyle of nonviolence, discarding distortions, owning up to my flaws, and forgiving myself were my answer to finding inner peace. I didn't have to fight anymore. There was nothing left that could be exposed or used as leverage against me. I knew that as long as I was authentic and my intentions were good, my foundation was unshakeable. The last bits of hypocrisy dissolved. I knew who I was, and I knew what I was here to do.

Enabling Sustainable Living

Later the same year, André and I opened a vegan, sugar- and gluten-free café in our hometown. At this time, the vegan revolution was in its early seedling period in Norway. With the café, we filled an unmet need for knowledge, resources, and support. Along with other vegan eateries, we were forced to close, even though we rocked five-star reviews. Then we created and hosted Green Food Fest—our own vegan, inspirational food festival—in 2017 and 2018.

André had always carried a dream of opening a vegan grocery store. He had long-term experience from managing other food store chains, and planning and executing events. I brought knowledge from the service, management, and social work fields. In the winter of 2019, he posted an inquiry online and we found our final team members, Erik Musum and Kristine Rykkelid. We knew Erik from co-organizing Gullroten, a vegan celebration and festival. He also has a band called Loud For The Animals that is dedicated to supporting animal activism. Whether it be educating children in Kenya or collaborating with others, Erik works to make the world fairer for everyone. His efforts spread optimism, inspiration, and hope, and have created opportunities for people to come together. Kristine made her appearance online. She's a natural-born adventurer with a passion for innovation and personal growth, and a deep love for nature preservation. She loves to challenge the status quo and contribute new solutions inspired by other continents. She grows some of her own food, and one day we'll publish her cookbook of epic vegan recipes collected from all around the globe! We all met up online and found similarities in our values, dreams, and viewpoints. We decided Greenseed Norge AS would be more than just the initial creators of Norway's first vegan food store chain. We wanted to work in vegan, sustainable concept development. I was ecstatic to have found a home where our ideas would come alive. We believe people are good and want to do good, if they have practical options.

> *Greenseed is a company where employees, partners, customers, and guests can come together and contribute to positive, sustainable change in our society, nationally and internationally.*—Erik Musum

Changing the World with 5XWIN

All of our creations are built with 5XWIN, our own two-part system that is both a philosophy and a tool for sustainable concept development. Compassion has taught me that we are all part of an indivisible whole, so when someone is hurt, we hurt collectively. The 5XWIN philosophy is based on principles of compassion, veganism, and kind living, which involve making choices that cause minimal harm. Furthermore, we believe that real sustainability can create collectively rewarding solutions such as have never previously existed. For an idea to be approved as sustainable, we check if the idea is beneficial to 1) the individual, 2) the community, 3) the animals, 4) nature, and 5) businesses. If the benefits are small, we scale them. Keep in mind that there is a distinct difference between causing harm and necessary unpleasantness. With 5XWIN, we all win!

We're always looking for ways to inspire, spread knowledge, simplify, optimize, and to enable people to be more sustainable in everyday life. We work as a catalyst for small businesses and entrepreneurs. We create platforms for different voices. Our first team project was *Make a Momentum,* a lifestyle blog based on co-creation that offers different perspectives on sustainable work and living. We feature posts about conscious living, self-growth, vegan recipes, and more. Vegan or not, anyone can become a co-creator because knowledge and the power to inspire positive change are alive in all of us. Different rhetorics and views resonate with different people. Joining forces with people you don't know on a personal level may seem risky, but everything is harder when you're alone. We use the power of collaboration to create a community of diversity, and this enables us to inspire the collective population on a larger scale. Amazing co-creators have already joined the movement on our various platforms and through our events.

> *I believe in dialogue, empathy, and understanding. I want to build bridges that bring us together as equals. I want an open world where your background doesn't dictate your opportunities.*—Kristine Rykkelid

We Are LOCO

According to a Norwegian newspaper, in 2019, the number of vegans in Norway had grown 80 percent in just the previous six years.[1] Orkla, a huge Norwegian food distributor, notes that their plant-based products increased in sales by 40 percent in 2020 compared to 2019. They think sales will double in 2021![2] NorgesGruppen, owner of multiple Norwegian food chains, seconds this optimism about the plant-based trend. I think we have just scratched the surface.

In September of 2020, we launched plans for LOCO, a full-range vegan grocery store chain. We will invite local producers, who face rejection from larger commercial chains, to make their full range of products available in LOCO stores. We're big on waste reduction and the circular economy. LOCO stores will provide free recipes and personal guidance. We'll host workshops to educate, support, and inspire people on their journeys. Products will be made widely available through technological solutions and collaborations that will enable local pick-up points.

> We let money control our options, and therefore our lives, far too much. As it is, society isn't supporting our best interests, and I want to do my part to change that.—André Gundersen

The cruelty in the world, whether real or in your mind, can trick you into victimhood, into feeling helpless. You're not helpless! Negative beliefs about your ability distract you from your purpose to achieve universal wellbeing. Honor your instincts to *feel*. Discomfort is your call to action. Compassion can be a tool for change or a weapon for destruction. We can all embrace the endless force of compassion for a more sustainable tomorrow.

Will you join us?

CHRIS HINES

Filmmaker and Animal Rights Activist

Vegan since 2014, Chris Hines has been involved in a number of campaigns and actions, working with organizations such as Viva!, Meat The Victims, Plant Based News, Anonymous for the Voiceless, DxE, and the Animal Save Movement. He has been interviewed on both TV and the radio on the subject of animal rights, given lectures at numerous UK colleges and universities, and spoken at events in the US and Europe. Chris is currently working on a feature-length documentary called *Taking Note*, which details the connection between music and animal rights and which features over one hundred musicians from across the globe. He is also the editor and founder of the online music and lifestyle website *HTF (Hit the Floor) Magazine*.

TO A NATION OF ANIMAL LOVERS

I have always considered myself an animal lover—from a young age, I was always fascinated by animals. I lived only a few minutes from the local zoo, for which my family had a season pass, so I'd spend a lot of time there reading the signs about the animals and copying information about them into an old textbook. We always had animals in the house as well, mainly cats, fish, and rodents; but in my teens, my brother and I became obsessed with reptiles, amphibians, and bugs, amassing a huge collection. When I left school, I went on to study an animal care course at the zoo for a year.

However, despite my good intentions toward animals, I was blissfully unaware of the effect I was having—not only on the animals I cared for, but also on the "invisible" animals I was consuming, wearing, and using. I say "invisible" in quotes because that's how they seem as I look back. I just didn't even think about them. Every day, I would sit in front of the TV and stuff the flesh and secretions of abused animals into my body. I would wear their skins as belts and shoes. Then I'd wash my face with products that had probably undergone horrific animal testing to be brought to market. The animals I kept in my home, whom I thought I was caring for, were really prisoners in boxes. The money I paid for them only ensured that more of their kind would live a life of captivity as well. My love of animals and my actions were totally hypocritical; I just didn't know it yet.

It was in 2002, when I bought an album called *Open Your Eyes* by the band Goldfinger, that things changed for me. The band had included a bonus video called "Meet Your Meat," which showed graphic footage of how we treat animals, soundtracked by an acoustic song called "Free Me":

So free me,
I just wanna feel what life should be.
I just want enough space to turn around,
and face the truth.
So free me.

The combination of these horrific images and powerful lyrics shook me to the core. I instantly became vegetarian. Many years later, after realizing the ethical holes in vegetarianism, I finally became a vegan in 2014, vowing to do everything I could to not contribute any further to animal suffering.

I'd watched all the films about what happens to animals, I'd done the research, but I needed to see things for myself. All we ever hear in the UK is: "It doesn't happen here." "England has the highest animal welfare in the world." "British farmers love their animals." But is there actually any truth to this?

I remember the first time I ever went to a slaughterhouse. It was a pig abattoir in Essex. Seeing the animals arrive and being able to interact with them, knowing that later that day they would be forced into a gas chamber to suffocate to death, were—needless to say—sobering experiences. We are fed time and time again claims of "high-welfare,"

"RSPCA-approved," "Red Tractor–approved," "free-range," etc., and the illusion that these standards are somehow "better" for the animals. Witnessing these animals just moments before their deaths rendered these labels false and misleading. These were scared animals who didn't want to die, and how they were "looked after" prior to this point was totally irrelevant. All that would have been needed to avoid their unnecessary deaths was if people had made some basic, habitual lifestyle changes.

Another slaughterhouse I visited had piles of cow and sheep skins—ready to be used for clothing or furniture. And once, along with some friends, I was even given a full tour of a family-run abattoir while desperately pleading that mercy be shown to a pig we met who was going to be slaughtered the next morning. He never saw his freedom. He was electrocuted, had his throat slit, and became someone's meal. We named him George.

Seeing animals face-to-face in the farms was a whole other experience.

You see images of undercover investigations and probably think these places are the worst of the worst; I can assure you they aren't. Most of what we see is, sadly, standard practice: thousands of chickens packed into sheds, dairy mothers struggling to stand after countless births, dead baby piglets found on the floor after being smashed into the ground because they weren't "up to standard," and lobsters and crabs with their claws tied together, thrown into piles to be sold and boiled alive. All these horrors I witnessed first-hand are commonplace and something I have seen time and time again.

I'll never forget seeing a mother pig in a farrowing crate for the first time. The crate was essentially a metal cage marginally larger than the pig, allowing her only to take a few steps forward and backward as she was unable to turn around. She was trapped. All she could do was sit or stand while staring blankly at the brick wall in front of her. Apparently, the purpose of these crates is to help protect baby pigs while they wean from their mothers, but it is not uncommon to find babies dead or dying next to mothers who stand there, unable to aid them. The pig would have been placed into one of these crates around five days before giving birth, then confined there for around twenty-eight days while her piglets were weaned. Nothing about this is humane; nothing about this is in her or her babies' best interest. I can remember so vividly just tearing up and looking into her eyes, knowing I was helpless to relieve her from that hell. All I saw was sorrow. As I returned home that night, all I could think about was how I was safe and warm in my bed while she remained, staring at that wall and waiting for it to end. Sadly, once she was freed from the crate, it would only be a matter of time before she was impregnated again and her confinement was repeated.

What we are doing to animals is no joke.

There is a quote commonly attributed to Gandhi: "The greatness of a nation and its moral progress can be judged by the way its animals are treated."

So what exactly does this say about the UK? To put things into perspective, just in the small area where I live in South West England, numerous horses are injured and killed from racing, badgers are culled in the thousands, foxes are torn apart by hunters, a factory ships live crabs over to China, and thousands upon thousands of sea creatures are ripped from the oceans—not only by local fishermen, but also by people who find it a "relaxing hobby." Pet shops buy and sell the lives of others for our entertainment, and every supermarket is lined with the cut-up dead bodies of sheep, cows, fish, pigs, chickens, and turkeys—all who wanted no more than to live their lives in peace.

And remember that zoo I used to love as a child? When you learn that most of the animals there will never see the wild, that more of these animals continue to be bred into captivity despite this, and that unwanted animals—such as the black rats, whose exhibit was deemed "not popular enough," and the peacocks, whose only crime was to nest too close to someone's backyard—are killed, it makes you question all the claims of "conservation."

All these abuses of life happen every second of every day, all across our country.

Something is incredibly wrong!

Animals are not just a collective group of nonhumans. They are not just objects, and they are certainly not just here for us to use and exploit at our will. Animals are individuals—mothers, fathers, and children; they make up families and communities. They are intelligent and sentient beings who experience this rock we call Earth in the same way as we do, each with their own unique life. We watch animals in awe; we want to spend time with them; and when close to them, we want to actively show them love. Yet we imprison them, destroy their homes, and exploit and use them in ways we never would each other—most of the time unconscious of what we are even doing.

We are lucky to live in a time when we no longer need to use animals for our own personal gain. Why, then, when we now have the choice to spare their lives, to eliminate their suffering and give them an opportunity to live in peace, do we not choose kindness?

The UK is one of the most vegan-friendly countries on the planet, and our Veganuary movement has inspired over a million people around the world to go vegan. Almost every chain restaurant now has vegan options on the menu, and nearly every supermarket has its own vegan range. Vegan-friendly cosmetics, toiletries, and clothing are everywhere. What is our excuse? We have none! Traditions, cultural norms, and personal pleasure should never be placed above someone's life—the most important and valuable thing we and all other beings will ever possess. Yet these are the excuses used every single day that enable the exploitation, abuse, and killing of animals to continue in every corner of our "Great Britain."

Every one of you reading this can make a choice today—right this second, in fact—to not play a part in other animals' suffering anymore, to be kind, to show compassion, just by making some simple life changes. You can choose not to wear or eat them, and you can refuse to support their exploitation. You can choose to align your actions with the morals you already hold, to respect that animals are here *with* us, not *for* us. We share this planet *together.* We are better than this, and we have the power to do better for them.

If we are to be the "Nation of Animal Lovers" we claim to be, we need to start acting like it, and that change starts with *you.* Please follow my lead, open your eyes, and help create a kinder world—for all of us.

NADIA MCKECHNIE

Vegan Community Organizer

Nadia McKechnie is the volunteer organizer of Tokyo Vegan, a community project that seeks to support the Tokyo vegan community in growing and connecting to the global vegan movement. Originally from London, UK, she works as a writer and narrator, and has lived in Tokyo for over thirty years.

VEGANISM IN JAPAN:
PRESENT CHALLENGES AND HOPES FOR THE FUTURE

My vegan activism largely revolves around Tokyo Vegan Meetup. The group had already been going for about eight years as a mainly English-speaking monthly event before I became its organizer in 2015. Around that time, there seemed to be a lot of new Japanese members. After I found a Japanese co-organizer, Saori Kondo, we made everything bilingual and set out to increase the number of events. Over the last six years, the group has tripled in membership to over 8,400 and expanded into a kind of vegan community project—Tokyo Vegan—with social and talk events (presently on Zoom), booths at festivals, and other activities. It's a kind of "portal" project, so we are happy to promote and share information about all kinds of other vegan-related projects. In 2019, we hosted over sixty events attended by more than 3,000 people. As many of the people coming to our events are not yet vegan, this has presented a great opportunity for outreach. I feel really fortunate to have met so many amazing vegan and vegan-interested people from Japan and around the world, and to have heard their stories. All this sounds really positive, but what is it actually like to be vegan in Japan these days?

The honest truth is that it's still challenging.

The first issue has to do with the nonavailability of vegan food. Japanese people traditionally consume very little animal protein; there seem to have been a number of reasons for this that are no longer very relevant to modern Japan, such as religious beliefs and a simple lack of arable land. Yet, today, there is an almost complete absence of foods and products labeled "vegan" or even "vegetarian" in restaurants and stores. In fact, just about every restaurant dish, takeout food, or packaged food often mixes in small amounts of animal ingredients. So while people certainly eat less meat in Japan than in many other countries, it can be hard to avoid animal ingredients.

Labeling laws in Japan are also somewhat vague, meaning that animal ingredients can be hidden in additives or flavorings. In many cases, the only way to check for sure is to actually call the company. Of course, there are some amazing vegan and vegan-friendly restaurants (especially in Tokyo) and an increasing number of products available online. But having to rely on social media and have the right apps is obviously not ideal when you are trying to get people to go vegan!

There are also several cultural issues that complicate matters.

In Japan, it is common to share dishes when eating out, and there is definitely the assumption that everyone will be able to eat everything that is offered. I recently discussed the reasons behind this with some of my Tokyo Vegan co-organizers. According to Yukari Iwamoto: "It's complicated. In Japan, we have two strong cultural norms surrounding food. The first one is *mottainai*—you should appreciate the food on the table, thus you should eat everything in order to avoid wasting any food or ingredients. The second one is *deru kui wa utareru*—literally meaning 'a stake sticking out gets hammered down.' Basically, in Japan, where harmony is highly valued, people are taught to eat everything, otherwise others will think of you as a troublemaker or someone who lacks cooperativeness." She went on to say: "The hardest part when I became vegan was being at a restaurant with someone else. When trying to ask for the possibilities to make something vegan, you get strange looks from both the people around you and staff members for causing trouble by making 'selfish' orders."

Kano Sekine agrees: "Yes, there are many situations, for example a work-related dinner, where it can be hard. Personally, I always tell people I'm vegan, but some of my friends are kind of in the closet. One reason for this is that Japanese students are not taught to exert their rights. People are expected to contribute to a work environment, where productivity comes first. Because people have low awareness of their own rights, advocacy movements, including animal advocacy, have not grown easily. I also know the feeling of being a 'closet vegan.' If you are considered selfish or weird for practicing a vegan lifestyle at work, you could lose the chance of promotion. I think it would help if activist groups like ours did more seminars at schools and more lobbying of lawmakers."

Saori Kondo had this to add: "I recently experienced how low acceptance still is when searching for a day nursery. I called some places to ask if they could accommodate us. None of them showed any understanding, or was even willing to let our son bring his own lunch. One place rejected us outright for even asking, and another place said they could accept him, but I would have to take him home while the other kids have lunch! One said that if he had allergies, they could accommodate him if we provided a doctor's certificate, but requests for a 'personal reason' could not be accepted. Another mentioned that they have to follow the menu provided by the government. It seems that if you have dietary restrictions because of religion or allergies, then schools and kindergartens cannot reject you. But if it's for an ethical reason, they can. Again, there's cultural background to this. People are still not willing to change what they perceive to be the traditional way. They do not want to make exceptions for fear of complaints from other parents, and above all, veganism is considered as a personal reason, and therefore 'selfish.'"

But although life in Japan can be challenging for vegans, our struggles pale into insignificance when we consider the situation of the animals. Something that I find most people are unaware of, both in Japan and overseas, is just how bad it is for the animals here. The truth is that in the 2020 World Animal Protection Index, Japan was ranked G (the lowest rank) in the category of "protecting farm animals." (Japan's overall ranking was E.)[3] I want to emphasize here that this is not because Japanese people are more unkind than anyone else. (In fact, as anyone who has visited Japan will attest, people are overwhelmingly kind.) It's just that there are few laws to protect farmed animals (or animals of any kind), so the systemic abuses—including the use of gestation crates and battery cages on factory farms—that are common in many countries carry on largely unchecked and unchallenged. The Humane League opened an office in Japan in 2017, and I asked Maho Uehara, its regional director, if there were any improvements in sight. She said: "The current law, Act on Welfare and Management of Animals, was enacted in 1973 and has been amended a few times. The law covers the animals raised and used for food production, yet there are no provisions for them. This is why it has been hard to address any animal abuse inflicted upon farmed animals. In 2020, some sentences related to livestock production were added, requiring local governments to strengthen cooperation with private organizations. Considering the history of the law, this was a huge step, but it still does very little for the animals. Awareness of animal issues among both businesses and the general population is extremely low."

But why exactly is awareness so low in Japan?

Certainly, there are the cultural issues that keep veganism in the shadows. But an even greater problem is the almost complete lack of information about animal issues in the media in Japanese. There are none of the documentaries, interviews, advertisements, celebrity quotes, newspaper articles, or even references to veganism that are now commonplace in countries where veganism is growing. Although the Japanese-language media is very slowly starting to cover the environmental dangers of animal agriculture, the animals themselves are still missing from the conversation. Recently, this has led to a number of "less-meat" products and menu items. But rather than being totally vegan, these contain smaller amounts of animal ingredients.

Add to this that the budgets of the fledgling animal rights groups in Japan are just a tiny fraction of those of similar groups overseas, and it's easy to understand why the number of vegans is still comparatively low. A recent survey by the website Vegewel put the percentage of vegans in

Japan at 2.1 percent,[4] but I would say that's extremely generous. It should be mentioned that the lack of funding is not a reflection of the Japanese groups' effectiveness. The work these groups—notably the Animal Rights Center Japan and PEACE—do is laying the foundation for real change in Japan. It's just that, as Saori-san pointed out: "It's difficult for groups to grow. Most people just don't join groups or financially support causes in Japan, and demonstrating publicly is frowned upon."

So where do we go from here?

Of course, there is social media. There are a few Japanese influencers who are starting to gain followers. We also have several new grassroots projects, a couple of fledgling farm sanctuaries, and a number of media-friendly restaurants, and Meat Free Monday All Japan recently opened the first-ever vegan food bank. These things are all helping to improve the visibility of veganism. The help of overseas campaigns is also invaluable. Veganism is a global movement and I hope Japan can connect to it more through sharing information and resources here and abroad.

And sometimes, hope for animals can present itself in unexpected ways.

The 2020 Tokyo Olympics, with its slogan "Unity in Diversity," definitely gave veganism in Japan a boost. In November 2019, the bipartisan Vege Council Japan, consisting of lawmakers, vegan-related groups, and vegan-related businesses, was set up to discuss the issue of the lack of vegan/vegetarian options and labeling ahead of the Olympics. Despite coronavirus concerns regarding the games, the council has continued to meet (Tokyo Vegan has been a part of this), and it's been beyond encouraging to see politicians engage with businesses, vegan groups, and the media, discussing how to make Japan more inclusive of vegans and even starting to broach issues such as climate change, health, and the animals. Given Japan's skill at innovation and its rich (although slightly forgotten) history of plant-based food, there seems to be a real possibility for change, even against the background of sociocultural issues and challenges.

In Japan, most discussions revolving around veganism are still focused on consumer habits and food products, and recently, climate change. Animal rights is still not an issue. It is my hope that by raising the visibility of veganism and making it easier to adopt veganism as a mainstream lifestyle choice, we will be able to open up a path to the start of real discussions about the way we collectively treat animals in Japan—and all over the world.

SHANKAR NARAYAN

Founder, Satvik Vegan Society (SVS)

Shankar Narayan is the founder of Satvik Vegan Society (SVS), the oldest Indian vegan organization with "vegan" in its name. SVS conducts the annual Satvik Vegan Festival (SVF) and International Vegan Festival (IVF, ranked among the most popular vegan events in the world). Shankar was an international councilor and regional coordinator (India and Southwest Asia) for the International Vegetarian Union (IVU) from 2006 to 2016. He currently lives in Sthitaprajna Vegan Forest, a forest regeneration project that he founded in 2009. Shankar is a member of the Vegan Task Force, which was constituted by the Food Safety and Standards Authority of India, the Ministry of Health and Family Welfare, and the government of India.

VEGAN, NATURALLY

Some people have compassion for—and empathy with—all beings. Some have compassion for only humans, others for only their own people, and yet others for no one at all. When you have compassion for all beings, you are a vegan, naturally. I am *vegan, naturally.*

When I was a child in school, teachers taught us that smoking and drinking were bad habits. I was wondering why they never included eating animals, which is more harmful than smoking and drinking. My young mind was questioning why taking the lives of animals and eating animal flesh were acceptable to society, yet smoking and drinking, which may harm the one doing these things but are less harmful compared to eating animals, were not okay. I had to wait for many years before I got answers to this predicament.

As a child, I suffered many types of abuse at the hands of my elders. I thought my suffering would not have existed if I had never been born. Perhaps this type of thinking influenced me in my decision to become *vegan, naturally,* later in my life. In 1989, when I read Mahatma Gandhi's autobiography, *The Story of My Experiments with Truth,* it was the final push and it was enough for me, a lacto-vegetarian by birth, to stop consuming milk. It was only in 2001 that I became a vegan after coming to know of The Vegan Society and the vegan movement.

I keep telling my listeners that "veganism is a journey, not a destination." The commonly accepted philosophy of veganism is that we can still lead happy and healthy lives when we don't eat or use animals, letting them live their lives without any interference from us. Learning to live without exploiting animals, to follow a different path compared to the majority of people, gives us an opportunity to think deeply, and critically evaluate all our actions and responses to the problems we face. It gives us the possibility to explore and find deeper meanings in our lives. It also reduces any negative impacts we may have on others' lives as well as our own.

In addition to nonviolence, these are further guiding principles to live by:

Simplicity: The rise in consumption by an ever-expanding population is becoming an increasingly huge burden on the earth. As some become rich and spend more, there are more and more people living in poverty. Even without a large population, we would do well with minimal needs and simpler living. The earth can't support such a huge consumer base while at the same time nonrenewable resources are being depleted day by day. To lead a happy and healthy life, we don't need to earn and spend without limits. We should be content with what we have. By moving away from the current socioeconomic system, which places such high priority on material gain and economic growth, we can learn to live with fewer resources. Not only will our lives become more peaceful, but the earth can regain its natural equilibrium, climate change can be reversed, and conflicts and wars can be reduced.

Truthfulness: Being truthful is one of our obligations to our fellow humans and animals. It is true that all living beings can sense pain. The truth is that every living being has the urge to live as long as possible. If we understand this truth, we will follow the path of truth and live without participating in violence against others.

Silence and Polite Language: Silence is a powerful language. We need to speak only when absolutely necessary, and in a polite manner. Actions speak louder than words, and silence is always golden. Silence can achieve what most words cannot. When we judiciously practice silence when appropriate, we can avoid many unpleasant situations and difficult conditions, and gain insights into a new way of being. Many saints sat in silence for months and years to reach enlightenment and salvation. Similarly, sitting in silence for at least a few minutes every day and for a longer duration at least once a week will bestow on us many benefits. When speaking is absolutely necessary, we should use polite and unhurtful language. Even if we are speaking an unpleasant truth, we should speak in such a way that conveys the message without hurting the feelings of the receiver.

Non-stealing: Stealing is taking another person's property without permission or legal right and not intending to return it. Stealing is not acceptable in our society and is punishable by various statutes. When we exploit and kill animals, we are stealing their lives, though most statutes do not recognize this as a crime. Ideally, an advanced civilization like ours should criminalize such acts. The growing exploitation of animals in our current industrial food systems also results in environmental damage and drastic depletion of our resources. The inefficiency and harm of using animals as a food source will affect future generations' abilities to live sustainably. We cannot continue to take the lives of our fellow animals, or take from Earth's natural resources as if they were inexhaustible.

Freedom: Freedom is the most precious gift one can give or take. The challenge for us as a society is to ensure that we retain freedom not only for ourselves, but for others, too. No individual should lose their fundamental rights—freedom of thought, speech, and movement— and the ability to live a healthy life without economic, social, or religious restrictions. Human society continually faces challenges, for our tendencies toward self-interest have led to inequalities, injustices, political conflicts, and personal entanglements. My dream is a world where every living being, whether human or nonhuman, is free.

* * *

In 2001, when I first turned to veganism, I felt alone. Most people, including family members, didn't understand my decision, and some even thought I was crazy. Up until about 2004, I did not come across a single vegan anywhere, either in Coastal Karnataka where I lived or in places where I traveled. No one knew of the concept of veganism. However, since then, there has been an exponential increase in the number of vegans in India. This is because vegan, alternative foods are becoming more and more available. For example, you now have soy, cashew, coconut, almond, and rice milks as substitutes for cattle milk.

By birth, we are all *vegans, naturally.* Through social conditioning, however, we adopted many harmful, unnatural practices along the way. Therefore, it is our duty as humans, with our intellectual power and evolutionary advantages, to first stop eating animals. Then, with the wisdom we gain from such a noble act, we must instill more peaceful practices that will not only empower ourselves and others, but also allow all beings to live and give our Earth the chance to heal.

DOREEN ROTHE

Campaigns and Volunteer Management,
Albert Schweitzer Foundation, Berlin

Doreen Rothe was born in East Germany in 1971. She came to Berlin in 1991 to study interpreting (English and Spanish). About a year later, she turned vegetarian and became active in an anti-vivisectionist organization. It took her eight more years to go vegan and some more to become a vegan activist. Subsequently, she joined the volunteer network Berlin-Vegan, which aims mainly to help people find their way around vegan Berlin and which established one of the world's largest vegan street festivals, the Veganes Sommerfest Berlin. By then, Doreen had been working for several years as a technical translator. When the opportunity came to work at the Albert Schweitzer Foundation, she accepted the position with great enthusiasm.

VEGANISM: A CHANGING WORLD

Some time ago, I took part in a flash mob under the motto, "I am vegan because. . . ." When I was preparing my poster, at first I could not decide what to write on it, as there are so many reasons for being vegan. In the end, I wrote, "Because it is the answer to some of the most urgent questions of our time."

We are living in a very critical time, perhaps the most critical in human history. Scientists have been warning us for decades. Their warnings are becoming increasingly desperate as the state of the environment has never been worse and is declining at a frightening rate. COVID-19 shows us once again just how vulnerable we are. The great majority of pandemics have had their origins in the raising of animals for food and the consumption of animals. The next catastrophe of this kind might be just around the corner—with unimaginable consequences. Also, the continuing overuse of antibiotics in factory farms escalates the risk of antibiotic resistance, which leads to the possibility of many people dying even from simple wounds as treatments lose their effectiveness.

But there are answers, one of the most effective of which is to consume fewer animal products or, even better, to live a vegan life. I think all vegans—and even vegetarians, come to think of it—hear questions along the lines of, "But what is there left for you to eat?" Well, I usually say, "Everything." I eat sausage and schnitzels, cream cakes and pancakes, raclette and pizza, ice cream and roulades—just made from plants. Living a vegan life does not mean self-denial or sacrifice. It is about replacing animal-sourced ingredients and animal products with plant-based alternatives and foods that do not cause suffering. Hopefully, one day, animal products will become obsolete.

The other day, my colleagues and I were talking about how we came to be animal rights activists and vegans. And when I told them I had turned vegan in 2001, they asked me how hard it had been back then. Being vegan in 2001 compared to today was certainly harder. But then, these days I find it extremely easy, at least when one lives in the vegan capital of Germany! When I travel to smaller towns or more rural areas, sometimes I am still looked at strangely when I ask for vegan options in bakeries or at restaurants. And although the number of vegans in Germany reached about 2.6 million in 2020 (double the number from just 2016 and many times that from 2008, when there were fewer than 80,000),[5] I am often shocked that many people know so little about the horrible conditions in animal agriculture and all the negative effects it has on our lives and the environment—and seem not to care.

Germany is considered one of the countries with the best animal welfare laws in the world. But when you look at how animals raised for food live and die, you would hardly believe this. Germans like to consider themselves animal lovers. We do love our pets and spend lots of money on them. But when it comes to food, especially animal products, nothing can be cheap enough. And while almost everyone strongly opposes industrial farming, far fewer people are willing to pay more for their food. In fact, there are few countries in Europe in which less money is spent on food than in Germany, and this is not because Germans eat less. We just ignore the actual price the animals—and ultimately we—have to pay in the end.

Therefore, I am very often quite torn between being very elated by positive developments and being devastated by how slowly progress seems to happen. But all in all, over these past twenty years, things have changed a lot, and it has been great to be able to experience these changes first-hand. I have to say that Berlin has been a great place in which to watch all this happen.

In 2001, there was but one little all-vegan shop, and I admire the owner for the stamina and courage she had back then, when vegans were still mostly frowned upon. The first two or three vegan restaurants opened sometime around 2008; when you went to one of them, you knew everyone there. Today, we have around eighty such places, and almost all restaurants and cafés have some vegan options to offer. And when you visit one of the vegan restaurants, it is rare that you know any of the other patrons; that is a good sign. Vegan food can be found in every supermarket and discount store; all have special vegan-offer weeks and promote these products as being particularly healthy or good for the environment. Over the twenty years I have been living vegan, an incredible number of new products have come onto the market. These days, there is a plant-based alternative to almost every animal product.

I will admit that before first becoming vegetarian, I used to eat meat every day and I loved the taste and consistency of cheese. But now, I can enjoy eating the vegan versions of such things—without all the negative aspects of animal products. In addition to these "veganized" counterparts to foods of my earlier years, there are a whole lot of completely new products. And I have met more than one person who has said that since turning vegan, their cooking style has become far more varied. Today, we even have several all-vegan shops here in Berlin, including several stores of Europe's first all-vegan supermarket chain, Veganz. The other day, I read that one in every ten newly released products in Germany is vegan. It is particularly promising that almost all major food companies, including some of the most well-known traditional meat and sausage companies, now offer vegan products. They have recognized the sign of the times. And as it is their products that most customers buy, they contribute a lot to the perception of vegan food becoming more normal.

Another common question vegans hear is, "Why do you have to imitate animal products when you do not want to eat animals?" Well, why do we use alternative energy sources or alternatives to plastic bags? Or why do we live in houses when we do not want to live in caves? Everything is constantly changing and developing—it is the very basis of evolution. But when it comes to our eating habits, we find it incredibly hard to accept any changes. I think one of the main reasons for this is that eating is not just necessary for our survival but also linked with a lot of special emotions and memories of childhood, with warmth and comfort. However, I feel that people are realizing that moving away from using animals is the way it should be; we need a new future of food—one that is vegan.

I have the great privilege to be able to work full-time for an animal welfare/animal rights organization, the Albert Schweitzer Foundation. This gives me the opportunity to spend as much time as possible on something I regard as so important for our future. Albert Schweitzer's fundamental maxim was reverence for life. So we focus on the single greatest source of pain and death for animals: their exploitation and use as products and food sources. One main pillar of our strategy is working with enterprises and convincing them to offer more vegan alternatives and make them more easily available to customers. What I particularly like about the foundation is its pragmatic approach, always based on the latest scientific findings. While we very decidedly work to promote the vegan lifestyle as the most ethical solution, we also try to achieve as many real improvements as possible in the lives of the countless animals who are still suffering for human consumption and will unfortunately continue to suffer for the foreseeable future.

Currently, we are concentrating on broiler chickens. Europe alone is fattening and slaughtering 7.2 billion chickens year after year.[6] We, as well as several other European animal welfare organizations, participate in the Open Wing Alliance, which developed the European Chicken Commitment to raise the minimum standards for broiler chickens on a transnational scale. While the ultimate goal is to bring factory farming to an end, we see it as a duty to move in a positive direction and reduce the suffering of these animals as much as we can. This Europe-wide—even global—approach is particularly effective, as it helps companies that are raising their standards not become disadvantaged in international competition as well as increases pressure on those lagging behind. We gain confidence in our approach from the way things are developing. I am very happy that our work is being acknowledged by Animal Charity Evaluators, which designated the Albert Schweitzer Foundation as a 2020 Top Charity for the third year in a row.[7]

Global problems concern us all, so we have to tackle them together. We are so much stronger together than alone. It feels wonderful to join forces with people from all corners of the world in the fight for something so important and to feel that strong kinship with them. This kinship among vegans and animal rights activists is something I particularly cherish. And it is not just about animal rights. Most vegans I know also have a very pronounced sense of justice in general and try to do as little harm as possible in their daily lives.

By the way, vegans are not enemies of farmers. On the contrary! We are not fighting them or agriculture. Agriculture is essential for all of us. But we are looking for another kind of agriculture—one that doesn't exploit animals, the environment, or people.

As humans, we are in the unique position to be able to reduce the amount of suffering and increase the amount of happiness in the world. As I said, we are living in unprecedented times. Never before has it been more urgent for us to act together for a better world, and never before has it been easier. So let us get together and make the world a better place to live for humans and nonhuman animals alike.

ORI SHAVIT

Food Journalist and Vegan Influencer

Ori Shavit is a food journalist and restaurant critic who used to eat everything until she became vegan about a decade ago. Since then, she has become one of the leaders of the most significant culinary revolution to have taken place in Israel in recent years. She is the founder of the blog *Vegans On Top*, regularly collaborates with leading food companies in Israel, develops recipes, leads cooking workshops, and gives talks on plant-based nutrition and the vegan lifestyle around the world. Ori also founded the successful vegan pop-up restaurant Miss Kaplan that operated in Tel Aviv. She is author of the best-selling cookbook *My Vegan Kitchen*, which has already sold twenty-five thousand copies in Israel. Her second cookbook, *Vegan Celebration*, was released in February of 2021.

THE ISRAELI FOOD REVOLUTION

It happened toward the end of 2011. I sat down with a friend at a well-known café in the center of Tel Aviv, and since I did not see anything vegan on the menu, I consulted with the waitress as to what I, newly vegan in those days, could order. She looked at me, confused, hesitated for a moment, then asked me, "Wait, you don't eat cheese, *too*?"

Only a decade has passed since the days when even in the most culinary and up-to-date city in Israel, not only did restaurants not offer vegan dishes at all, but many people hardly knew what veganism was. Ten years in which there was nothing short of a food revolution in Israel, which changed the way many Israelis eat and make their dietary choices. A revolution that, although it begins on a plate, is also economic, social, and ethical in nature, whose effects are evident in many areas of the Israeli way of life.

Today, Israel is a vegan power nation. It is considered the country with the highest percentage of vegans and vegetarians in the world (about 5 percent of Israelis declare themselves vegan and another 8 percent vegetarian), and it has a particularly high percentage of flexitarians. About 35 percent of Israelis claim to have reduced their animal consumption in recent years. As of the time I am writing these words, more than one hundred companies and projects are offering, producing, and developing a large variety of alternatives to animal products, and the volume of plant-based products already being sold in market chains is constantly expanding. Advertisements promoting vegan products like vegan milk and vegan burgers are broadcast on prime-time TV, and almost all national restaurant and coffee chains offer customers a wide selection of vegan dishes that are clearly marked on the menu. Even in the dining rooms of the Israeli army, a growing selection of vegan dishes is served, in light of the number of vegan soldiers having increased significantly in recent years. When you look back and see how fast and to what extent this change has taken place, it is impossible to call it anything other than a revolution.

The fact that such a significant revolution took place in Israel is not accidental; it stems from a unique mix of characteristics that allowed the vegan trend to flourish in Israel. Israel is a young country built by immigrants from all around the world, who came with their unique cultures and cuisines. The result is a mix of different cooking traditions, which has made Israelis more flexible in their way of eating rather than sticking to one traditional cuisine with fixed and strict rules. This is probably part of what contributed to the well-known Israeli love for innovation and openness to new experiences. It is not for nothing that Israel is called the "start-up nation," and it is not surprising that the desire to innovate is expressed on the plate as well as elsewhere. In terms of diet, Israel's geographic location probably also made it an ideal, fertile ground for veganism: the Mediterranean diet is based on plenty of fresh vegetables and fruits, is rich in grains and legumes and generous with its use of olive oil, so the average Israeli diet already contains quite a few vegan foods. Even Israel's national dishes—hummus and falafel—are originally vegan, so no matter where you are across the country, you will always have something to eat.

You can add to all of this two more interesting facts: The first concerns Jewish kosher laws, which are familiar to anyone living in the country, even if they are not religious. The very idea of avoiding certain foods, separating foods, and labeling products as "dairy," "meat," or "Parve" (not containing milk or meat) is not foreign to the Israeli public and increases tolerance of dietary restrictions—including vegan diets— in the kitchen. The fact that Israel has a huge crowd of kosher observers significantly increases the target audience for vegan foods. The Jewish religion allows these products marked as "Parve" to be eaten at any time, even with meat and milk, thus greatly increasing their demand. The second parameter that has helped the success of veganism in Israel greatly is the country's size: Israel is a tiny state about the size of New Jersey, so when a certain trend gains momentum, it spreads very quickly. When information about the vegan lifestyle started popping up, especially through activists' use of the rising power of social media networks, it was impossible to remain ignorant of it. In this way, millions of Israelis were exposed to the important reasons for choosing veganism: reducing harm to animals, maintaining health, and protecting the environment. Indeed, many people have decided to make a change, becoming vegan or at least reducing their consumption of animal products.

I was one of these people; only, for me, it was a more dramatic upheaval than just a decision to change my diet. In those days, I was a food journalist and restaurant critic at the leading gastronomy magazine in Israel, and most of my work was, naturally, eating—eating everything. Beyond the profession, I had a deep passion for and a genuine interest in food of all kinds, accompanied by a hedonistic lifestyle that included dining in many restaurants, sitting in bars, and covering everything taking place in the fascinating Israeli food scene. Back then, I even had an ideology that placed supreme value on deliciousness and according to which avoiding certain types of food was a disgrace. In other words, I was the furthest away from veganism that you can imagine, and I also made a living from it. I did not see any change on the horizon, nor did I want any.

But then I went on a date with a guy who, after five seconds, turned out to be vegan. I immediately knew it was a waste of time because there was no chance I could associate with someone so different from me, a guy I could not even go out to eat with! On the other hand, I was already on a date with him and, like a good journalist, decided to make good use of the time and interrogate him about his strange decision to give up lots of delicious foods. This conversation opened a door for me to a world I did not know and had never researched. Especially as a food journalist, I was shocked to find out how ignorant I was about different aspects of the food industry; and not only did I not know many things about it, but there were so many questions I had never asked. Basic information such as how milk and eggs are produced and what these industries do to animals had never come to my mind, partly because I had never bothered to learn about these issues. This turmoil led me to research the subject more deeply, and I quickly realized that if I did not want to continue taking part in and promoting the horrible cruelties that I was exposed to, then I had no choice but to go vegan.

In my case, it was a revolution no less great than the one that Israel was going through. I had to resign from my dream job because in those days, there was nothing vegan to write about in a reputable gastronomy magazine. I had to reinvent myself, but I did not want to *become* someone else. I perceived vegans as weird, lonely fringe people who ate sprouts in the dark. As a hedonistic Tel Avivian who was used to sitting in a different restaurant every night, I was not ready to become one of "them"! I decided to prove that it could be done differently—that I could be vegan but continue to be who I was, eat delicious food, hang out in restaurants, and show that anyone could enjoy life as a vegan. I wanted to keep writing about food, and within two months, the blog *Vegans On Top* (Hebrew for "vegan girls have more fun") was up and running. I had planned to document my transition to veganism and share what I learned along the way, but never in my wildest dreams could I imagine that this would be the beginning of a successful and even international career that would take me farther than I had dreamed possible.

Today, most of my work is related to the promotion of vegan cuisine and culture in Israel. I lead vegan cooking workshops, the demand for which has grown especially since the outbreak of the coronavirus pandemic and as more people desire to eat healthy and sustainable food. I develop recipes for my blog and am the author of best-selling vegan cookbooks. I advise restaurants and food manufacturers in their development of vegan dishes and products. My two TEDx talks have helped me convey my message globally, and I speak about veganism around the world. I have been interviewed in the media and have taken part in a variety of activities that helped uncover information about the implications of our diets for us and the world around us.

I am often asked for the best tip that I can give to someone who has realized how important it is to change their eating habits but who is having a lot of difficulties. I know this predicament from experience, for I, too, thought that switching to a plant-based diet would be very difficult and that I would have to purchase expensive ingredients and spend more time in the kitchen, only to still be hungry at the end of the day. The reality, especially today, is much different. With proper organization and a short adaptation process, most people find that it is much easier and simpler than they thought. I think the most important thing you need when you enter the kitchen is not special equipment or certain ingredients, but rather a smile. When you enter the kitchen, do so with joy and curiosity from a desire to learn new recipes, get to know new ingredients, and prepare dishes you did not know. Look at the process of getting to know vegan cuisine as an adventure, as recreation time in a playground you have not yet entered, and the results will be happy and delicious. If you keep thinking about what you have taken off your plate, what you're missing, and how hard it is, chances are your food will be just as depressing.

The second most important thing you need to have is support. Despite the huge increase in the number of vegans around the world, veganism is still not widespread, and those who are vegan are usually the minority in the area in which they live. Support and help from good contacts and experienced vegans will be especially beneficial in the beginning, as from them you get answers to all the questions that arise about nutrition, cooking, fitness, children, and more. That is exactly why an international project called Challenge 22 has been established in Israel, providing exactly this type of support to new vegans and those interested in veganism. The challenge is free and takes place online in a supportive and friendly atmosphere in a closed Facebook group, with contributions from experienced mentors in all fields—dietitians and cooks, parents, athletes, and veteran vegans. The challenge is run in different languages around the world and I highly recommend you join.

MARLY WINCKLER

Chair, International Vegetarian Union (IVU)

Marly Winckler, sociologist, is the translator of more than sixty books, including *Animal Liberation* by Peter Singer. Vegetarian since 1983 and vegan since 1995, she created Sitio Vegetariano, the first webpage on vegetarianism in Portuguese, as well as veg-brasil and veg-latina (now ivu-latina), the first discussion lists about vegetarianism in Portuguese and Spanish. Marly served as Latin American and Caribbean Coordinator of the International Vegetarian Union (IVU) from 2000 to 2013, and was president and founder of the Brazilian Vegetarian Society (SVB) from 2003 to 2015. Marly was the IVU chair from 2011 to 2014 and has held the same position from 2018 to the present. She lives in the beautiful island city of Florianópolis, where she organized the 36th IVU World Vegetarian Congress in 2004.

EXPEDITION OF A VEGAN TO THE HEART OF THE AMAZON

Undertaking an expedition to the Amazon from the south of Brazil where I live is not the easiest task, nor the cheapest. It can cost more than going to Europe. In 2014, I made the fifteen-hour trip from Florianópolis to Faro, a city in the state of Pará, which would serve as our headquarters. It was a journey of more than 4,500 kilometers. We were a group of three vegans interested in observing eating habits, and collecting information and images about the devastation of the forest, the relationship between people and animals, and other local peculiarities. The trip was twelve days in all, including visits to Parintins, Faro, surrounding riverside communities such as Nhamumdá, and other islands and villages.

The Dimensions of the Amazon

The Amazon is a huge region. It extends 3,500 kilometers from the Andes Mountains to the Atlantic coast and covers an area of 7 million square kilometers, representing two-thirds of the world's tropical forests. In addition to Brazil, it covers eight other countries: Bolivia, Colombia, Ecuador, Guyana, French Guiana, Peru, Suriname, and Venezuela. It spans nine Brazilian states, equivalent to an area about the size of the entire US. It occupies 60 percent of the Brazilian territory and is home to 15 percent of all living species in the world. The Brazilian Amazon has a population of about 30 million. The Amazon is home to approximately 180 different indigenous tribes, adding up to a population of approximately 200,000. Another 70 to 100 groups live in isolation. Until 1970, less than 2 percent of the Amazon area had been deforested. Today, almost 20 percent has already been cut down, and the destruction process continues to increase on a large scale. According to the Brazilian government, at least 80 percent of deforested areas are used for livestock and another 10 percent for the cultivation of soy, which serves as animal feed.

I already knew the "other side" of the Amazon—Mato Grosso and Rondônia—and had seen my own state, Santa Catarina, being devastated to open up areas for livestock and to grow the soy and corn used mostly for feed. So deforestation issues were not entirely new to me. While there are regional peculiarities, deforestation methods are similar across the country, with increased rates of destruction made possible with the help of the chainsaw.

Riverside Populations

We did not visit large units of soy or cattle production responsible for the greatest amounts of deforestation. We focused on riverside populations, visiting some small properties in the Faro region. There is a desire among the population to be, so to speak, a livestock farmer. Thus, many residents of towns and cities, despite already having a job, try to buy an area of land and begin its "creation." There are laws that regulate how much of the property can be cleared, but this is circumvented most of the time, often illegally, with practically no inspection. Then an "ant's work" is done, step by step and almost invisibly: The main trees in a small area of forest are cut down and set on fire. Corn or beans are immediately planted, followed shortly after by the planting of grass for cattle to graze on. These small properties, with an average of one hundred to two hundred heads of cattle, provide savings for their owners. Others live off cattle ranging only, but it is a culture that brings few financial benefits. When the oxen are ready for slaughter, they are taken to the municipal slaughterhouse, and what was illegal becomes legal. The oxen are slaughtered, and the meat is sold right there.

It is worth remembering that access to these cities is by river. In fact, most of these communities and villages have only a few hundred inhabitants; few of them reach a thousand. One of the largest towns in the region, Faro, founded in 1768, has only seven thousand inhabitants. There are no roads—yet—in this region, which ends up being a blessing because when roads are built, the degree of forest destruction increases exponentially. However, as a rule, the population would like to have roads and sees occupation as necessary. The soil of the Amazon is poor, and where cattle are raised, the land is useless for other agricultural activities. As you often hear over there, "Where the ox treads, you don't plant."

What We Ate

In Manaus, capital of the state of Amazonas, we had no difficulty feeding ourselves. There were vegetarian restaurants, always with vegan options. As a rule, breakfast at hotels had a good supply of fruit, and made-on-the-spot tapioca (a kind of starch) pancakes were highlighted, stuffed with freshly grated coconut and fruit if we were lucky. Juices and açaí were abundant. There is a good custom in the northern and northeastern regions of the country of eating roots for breakfast. These include cassava and yam, in addition to tapioca. And they are delicious! In Faro, we ate all meals in a pension (boarding house), where we could eat rice and beans (the salvation of vegans), braised cabbage, and salads generally consisting of lettuce, tomato, onion, cabbage, and other leaves. There were almost always boiled or fried potatoes and sautéed vegetables. And a lot of delicious cupuaçu juice was made to order.

What People Eat

Anyone who comes from abroad would imagine that riverside communities eat a lot of fish and game meat. But that's not really true nowadays. Fish are becoming scarce in the Amazon. This is because industrial fishing boats "sweep" rivers, removing everything that lies ahead. Game animals who typically would live near these communities have either already been killed or have withdrawn deep into the woods. So to my surprise, I found that what these people eat is chicken, which comes from the state where I live, Santa Catarina. It arrives by boat, frozen, along with some vegetables (tomatoes and onions mainly) and industrialized products in general.

Traditionally, the food of the riverside people was composed of fish and manioc, but it has been gradually replaced by industrialized foods. This is the result of, among other factors, a cultural change promoted by television that reaches even the most hidden corners of the Amazon. The typical foods of the forest have been replaced by agricultural foods based on meat, corn, soybean, sugar cane, and so on. It is a matter of opportunity: people will eat chicken and instant noodles if these foods are more affordable. Important foods for indigenous peoples, on the other hand, include fish and game meat, as well as cassava, sweet potatoes, corn, bananas, and pineapples. Some indigenous peoples do not eat red meat. But even these peoples have been changing their diets.

Visit to the Municipal Slaughterhouse

We contacted the city health inspector, who informed us that he had interdicted the municipal slaughterhouse from operating for hygiene violations. There was even a commission from the state capital, Belém, that ratified the interdiction. But as there was no alternative and the situation was the same in the nearest cities, they allowed the activity to continue. We paid a visit to the municipal slaughterhouse of Parintins on a day when there was no slaughter (every other day, eighty to two hundred oxen were killed). We entered the enclosure—a huge pavilion where the slaughter happened. The air was heavy, the smell strong and nauseating. Slaughter and cutting instruments were hung or positioned to do the job. Normally, the animals enter one by one through an opening from an adjacent corral where others "wait their turn." As soon as they enter, they each receive a blow to the head with an ax or sledgehammer and are immediately lifted by a hind leg for bleeding. Then they are dropped on the floor, where they are left in a pool of blood, feces, and vomit while being slaughtered. Many times, the ox is still alive during this process!

The scene in the corral was unpleasant. The animals, having spent the night without water and food, were scared, unable to understand what was happening. Their eyes were bloodshot. There were many buffalo, and we learned they were the ones who resisted the most. They had already gone through the stress of being removed from the pastures where they had lived. You can imagine how they resisted getting on boats to be transported by river. As they screamed, several men pushed them with sharp instruments, and the animals were beaten to move forward. While sailing on the river, we could see these violent scenes.

According to health regulations, blood and waste cannot be released into the river. Therefore, at the slaughterhouse, there was a pool full of blood, and large shovels were used to move the liquid so it didn't clot. This was one of the most disgusting scenes I had ever witnessed, and I almost threw up from the horrible smell that came from the material, which ended up going to the river anyway because it was considered not economical to treat it in any other way. In the corral, the oxen were crammed together; with so many being in a small space, they were "glued" to each other, unable to sit or turn around. On walkways built on the sides of the corral, the butchers who had come to buy their products chose the oxen to be slaughtered. And they were not depressed, as we would be; they spoke loudly and laughed all the time. Is this a psychological mechanism to mask what was really being done there?

And Now?

Much of the solution to deforestation in the Amazon is linked to changes in eating habits and land occupation. If vegetarianism is encouraged and adopted as a public policy, the situation could change dramatically, and with great results. However, there are currently no signs that this would happen in the short or medium term. Even organizations concerned with conservation that have operated in the region for decades have only recently started to touch on food issues, if at all. So unless critical concerns are raised about the severe damages resulting from deforestation and the livestock industry, I cannot have any hope that what is happening in the Amazon can be reversed.

The case of Brazil reflects the global situation: cattle use 40 percent of the planet's agricultural land. In Brazil, cattle occupy 200 million hectares and agriculture takes up 80 million. There are more than 200 million head of cattle. The country has more oxen than people. The area destined for livestock will increase to 300 million hectares occupied by 400 million animals in twenty-five to thirty years if nothing is done—and that will be the end of the Amazon and the Cerrado (another Brazilian biome that suffers the same impacts).

The last great natural area on Earth is being consumed by a combination of meat and soy. We are destroying the Amazon without even knowing it. Will we be able to save the Amazon? As Thomas More says at the end of *Utopia*, "I rather wish than hope."

SECTION THREE
Activism

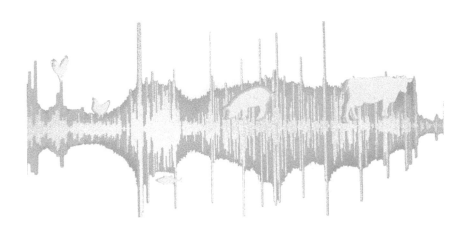

HOPE BOHANEC

Activist, Author, Podcaster

Hope Bohanec has been active in animal protection and environmental activism for thirty years and has published the book *The Ultimate Betrayal: Is There Happy Meat?* She is the projects manager of the national nonprofit United Poultry Concerns (UPC), the host of UPC's *Hope for the Animals Podcast*, and the executive director of Compassionate Living, a California-based vegan advocacy organization. Over the last three decades, Hope has given countless presentations, written innumerable articles, and organized hundreds of events, including UPC's annual Conscious Eating Conference and the Sonoma County VegFest.

THIRTY YEARS OF RADICAL COMPASSION

The bloody, severed bear paw on the hood of my car was sending panic through my workplace. I came out to the parking lot of the natural foods store to investigate. I knew immediately who had put that poor animal's severed paw on my car. This intimidation tactic was an attempt by the small traveling circus in town to frighten me. It didn't. But it certainly scared my co-workers, who had called the police and were swarming around my vehicle.

With the group SPAR (Sonoma People for Animal Rights), I had been organizing protests against all the small traveling circuses that came through Sonoma County, California, in the summers of the 1990s, and we were gaining sympathy and media attention. Any circus that dared to come to Sonoma County was surrounded by brave activists who would videotape its every move with cameras as big as toasters on their shoulders. We called animal cruelty violations into the local Humane Society and would leaflet attendees at every show, sometimes for two or three shows a day. Attendance went down every year, and after several years, the circuses started skipping Sonoma County on their tours of Northern California.

Just a few decades later, in the US, like in many other parts of the world, wild animals are no longer dragged around the country in circuses, no longer beaten and starved to perform tricks. Because of dedicated activists who continued this fight into the 2000s, we won that battle. Had you told me back then—when I was holding my sign that read, "The Circus Is No Fun for Animals"—that circuses would no longer have wild animals in just twenty-five years, I would not have believed it. Things can change very quickly, especially when we have love and compassion on our side.

Looking back, I'm rather amazed I wasn't more intimidated by the bear paw incident. But it wasn't the first time someone had tried to upset me or deter me from activism. I had been spat on during anti-fur protests and had had bottles and trash thrown at me while educating about animals suffering in laboratories. I had been threatened at rodeo protests to be run over with giant pickup trucks and—more often—had had mean and snarky remarks howled at me whenever I was simply asking for compassion for animals. These incidents left no scars, just a tougher skin and a calloused persistence. My resolve was—and still is—unbreakable, and some verbal and psychological abuse is nothing compared to what the animals endure day after day, year after year, in animal industries. But it does take a certain courage to be an activist. I didn't realize it then, but activists need not only perseverance but also a good degree of bravery to persist.

I worked at that natural foods store for fourteen years, but whenever someone asked me what I did, I said I was an animal rights activist, because that was my passion and what occupied my heart and mind almost every waking hour. I eventually found employment with animal rights nonprofits so that my full attention could be focused on creating a compassionate, vegan world. When I walked away from the natural foods market, that was the last time I had health insurance and financial security, but I knew that I was fulfilling my destiny to be a warrior for animals. For whatever reason, I had the spirit and temperament to endure watching horrifying videos of torturous cruelty and hearing about sickening abuses every day. Not everyone has the strength to do it. But I did, so I knew I *must*.

Over the last three decades, I have organized outreach tables, vegan potlucks, protests, film showings, vegan food samplings, and video outreach events. I have organized and given presentations at conferences and festivals, and have written a well-received book. In the last decade, I have worked for the highly respected national nonprofit United Poultry Concerns (UPC) and helped organize campaigns like UPC's International Respect for Chickens Day. When the pandemic hit and the world was suddenly on lockdown, I sat at home, stunned that all my outreach events had been brought to a standstill. But the breeding and killing of farmed animals did not stop, so I adapted and started a podcast; I have single-handedly recorded, edited, and produced over twenty *Hope for the Animals Podcast* episodes.

What Will You Be When You Grow Up?

From a very young age, I had a deep empathy and love for animals and a longing to help them. When I was a child, I had pictures of animals pinned up all around my room. When people would ask me what I wanted to be when I grew up, I would say that I was going to work with animals. I didn't know exactly what that would look like, but through my teens, my rebellious leanings and strong opinions drew me to activism.

My first activist inspiration came from Greenpeace back in the 1980s. I was moved by their dangerous and daring actions, which I saw on television, and my first job was with an East Coast Greenpeace chapter right after I'd graduated from high school. I soon heard about the plight of the ancient redwood trees being cut down in Northern California, and having always wanted to go to California, I packed up my car and headed west—with my cat on my lap for the entire drive. The radical, hardcore, direct-action activism of Earth First! was incredibly inspiring to me, and I was soon heading out early on damp, foggy mornings to do "lock-downs," blocking the logging roads with our bodies and various devices that made it difficult to move us, and "tree sits," whereby we would identify trees in danger of being cut down, and ascend these ancient giants with ropes and harnesses in the darkness of night. We built small wooden platforms and lived as high as 150 feet off the ground to protect these incredible forests. For a three-month period, I called the forest my home, living in a large hammock tied between four trees. My body ached from being unable to stand up the entire time, and answering the call of nature in a bucket 80 feet up in the air is something I will never forget. The danger was real, and sadly, a dear friend of mine, Beth O'Brien, fell 150 feet from a tree sit and died. This selfless activism I took part in in my early twenties with other courageous people affirmed the calling that I had long been feeling: I would be an activist for the rest of my life.

During my time with Earth First! I was reading and learning about the suffering of farmed animals. I was already vegan, but the cows, chickens, pigs, turkeys—they were calling me. They seemed to be the ultimate underdogs—innocent and defenseless, and in more misery and anguish than any other animals on Earth. At the time, there were very few people speaking out for them. In the early 1990s, I moved to the San Francisco Bay Area and brought the blockading tactics I had learned from Earth First! to local animal rights activism. I soon bonded with a small group of gutsy vegans. We blockaded slaughterhouses; we would shut down production with our necks in bike locks connected to the gates and our arms locked in cement-filled tubes and barrels. Some activists dangled precariously on wooden tripods, 20 feet in the air, all to make a statement and get media attention. However, we didn't have social media or the Internet, so it was difficult to tell our stories and control the narrative. This type of activism was high-risk and tough to sustain, with numerous arrests incurring large expenses. My activism eventually evolved into the vegan education and advocacy I do today, but my current dedication was seeded by my radical roots in the 1990s.

Times They Are a-Changing

I feel blessed to have a perspective that comes from three decades of vegan and animal rights activism. The incredible progress is impressive, and I'm proud to have played a small part in the achievements. The sheer volume of vegan options in grocery stores and at restaurants has vastly improved. At the store, there used to be just one shelf of vegan alternative foods, and they were so-so in quality and taste. That is certainly not the case anymore. Whatever you are craving, there is likely a delicious vegan option available. Commercials on television for oat and almond milks, as well as the new vegan options in the fast food sector, are just a few of the hopeful signs that compassionate, plant-based foods are rapidly going mainstream.

However, I think that the biggest advancement is evident in people's awareness and attitude. When I started this work in the 1990s, people had hardly heard of the word "vegan." I often got blank stares and confused expressions as I tried to explain. If someone did know what the word meant, then there was almost assuredly a negative reaction. Whether it was a snarky remark, an attempt at a joke, or an outright insult, the retort to the revelation of my veganism was almost always negative.

This has changed dramatically. In the last decade, not only have increasing numbers of people come to know what veganism is, but their reactions have become no longer overwhelmingly negative. In fact, I would say that the most common response I hear now is something along the lines of, "Oh, I don't eat much meat," or, "We drink almond milk." What people are basically saying is that they acknowledge my veganism as a good thing and that they are striving to eat better. It's a remarkable improvement in attitude and acceptance. I don't think new vegans realize just how far we have come.

Hope for the Future

I am very hopeful about the future. The animal liberation movement has a huge advantage: people love animals. The natural response to a cute animal is adoration and affection, and the vast majority of people don't want to see animals suffer. When people see an animal in distress on the side of the road, they stop traffic and risk their own lives to help save him or her. I truly believe that the deeper, better part of our nature is *compassion*. As animal activists, we simply remind people of this innate compassion and show them that farmed animals are in no less need of rescue from distress. The science of findings that vegan diets greatly reduce the risk of disease and also reduce one's contribution to climate disruption is icing on the vegan cake.

It will be a slow process, as deeply held beliefs and traditions are hard to fracture, but the progress we have already made for animals over the last four decades is inspiring. We have seen amazing improvements to combat so many forms of oppression all over the world. Even though the struggle for human rights goes on, it's nonetheless heartening to think how far we have come for women, children, and minorities. But, of course, there is still much more work to do.

I do believe that we are in the middle of a global awakening of consciousness—a collective shift toward peace, nonviolence, and compassion, toward a future in which all sentient life on this planet will be treated with respect and reverence and allowed to live free of human-imposed suffering. We must hold this vision of a compassionate, vegan world in our hearts and in our actions, and we just might see big changes for animals in our lifetime. Indeed, we already have.

SHWETA BORGAONKAR
Social Justice Organizer

Shweta Borgaonkar is an animal rights activist from Pune, India. At the time of this essay, she is twenty years old, and her mission in life is to create a world where all animals are respected and treated as individuals. She started out volunteering at adoption camps for stray cats and dogs and joined a vegan activism group at the age of sixteen. She co-organized Pune's first Animal Liberation March in 2018 and the Pan-India Animal Liberation March in 2019. Shweta has also led training sessions to help activists become better organizers. She co-organized the Pune chapters of Direct Action Everywhere (DxE) and the Animal Save Movement. Currently, she is doing undergraduate work in the field of commerce and is an aspiring law student.

HOW I BECAME A VOICE FOR THE ANIMALS

I grew up in a city with not many animals around. Growing up with a lack of interaction with animals, I was scared of them. This changed when Girija, a street dog, came into my life. In the beginning, I used to be so scared of her that I would walk on the edge of the road to avoid being in close proximity to her. But slowly, with her beautiful black eyes and wagging tail, she made my fear go away and became my best friend. This was the first time I had connected with a nonhuman animal so deeply. Something inside of me loved her unconditionally and she loved *me* back unconditionally.

One day, I went to class and everyone told me that Girija was no more. She had been hit and killed by a vehicle. I was devastated. I somehow controlled my tears in class. The thought that one day Girija wouldn't be in my life had never entered my mind. But I knew she didn't deserve to die like this. She deserved a safe home with a loving family.

She deserved to live in a world where everyone respected her, where she had access to medical care and food, and where her life was valued. As Girija left my life, she left me with a purpose in life—to create that world for her fellow Earthlings.

I joined a group called Pet Voices and started volunteering at adoption camps to help animals find good homes. But I knew that I wanted to do much more, something that would have a greater impact for animals. One day, in my tenth-grade class, we were discussing how it is standard practice, after a mother cow gives birth, to sell her colostrum. The colostrum is the thick initial milk produced by the cow within twenty-four hours of giving birth. It provides essential antibodies, proteins, and vitamins for her calf. In India, colostrum is sold to make *kharvas*, a pudding-like dessert made by steaming colostrum and sugar. Our teacher told us about an NGO (nongovernmental organization) that pays dairy farmers to let the calves drink the colostrum instead of selling it. She told our class that when we grew up, we should support such causes. This got me thinking about the morality of consuming *kharvas*. The idea of *letting* a calf drink their mother's milk bothered me. The word *let* means "to allow." Why would a calf need permission from anyone to drink their own mother's milk, especially within twenty-four hours of being born? That very moment, I decided I would never eat *kharvas* again. I couldn't possibly consume something that steals a baby's right to have their mother's milk. After a few months, I came across a post on Instagram that explained how egg-laying hens are killed after two to three years, when they stop producing high numbers of eggs. That's when I quit eating eggs. Similarly, I came across a post about how cows in the dairy industry are forcefully impregnated, then killed after a few years. I was shocked to learn that cows actually have to be pregnant in order to produce milk. It was hard giving up cheese and ice cream at first, but it was in no way comparable to the pain and suffering of animals in dairy farms. I realized that exploitation begins the moment we take away the purpose of an animal's life and impose *our* own purpose on that life, no matter how "humanely" the animal is treated.

The oppression of nonhuman animals is so normalized that most of society is unaware of their plight. So many of us are kindhearted people but have never had the opportunity to know about these issues or question the status quo. I was lucky to find an amazing activist group in Pune, and very soon afterward, I started organizing outreach events. Less than a year into my activism, I organized my first protest outside a major seafood restaurant in the city. I had forgotten about my materialistic dreams of being rich and owning a sea-facing house with an infinity pool. Instead, I became a minimalist, and spreading the vegan message became my only focus.

In 2018, my friends Suchitra and Sanjeev invited me to attend the Animal Liberation Conference in Berkeley, California. This is an annual event organized by Direct Action Everywhere, and it's a literal heaven for vegan activists. The week-long event, attended by hundreds of activists from all over the world, included life-changing trainings by the best activists, lip-smacking vegan food, and public demonstrations and vigils. On the last day of the ALC, activists went inside a Whole Foods chicken supplier farm and rescued thirty-seven birds in broad daylight. The activists said that the conditions in these factory farms clearly violated animal cruelty laws and that if one had the right to rescue a dog from a hot car, then one also had the right to rescue these birds, who were clearly dehydrated and some of whom had even cannibalized each other out of starvation. Some activists, refusing to leave until all the animals were released and given sanctuary, were arrested by the police. The action taken by the activists to save these chickens was all over the news and completely changed the way I saw the animal rights movement.

I learned two very important things from that action. First, it is important to have a clear path to your goal. Our movement needs to develop strategies that will take us closer to the goal of animal liberation. The focus of my activism prior to this action had been fixed on the goal of motivating the greatest number of people possible to go vegan. But I had never thought about how these vegans would help liberate all the animals who are used and abused. Maybe making more people go vegan should not be the only strategy we use. Secondly, it took hundreds of activists, dozens of very skilled organizers, research, and months of training to save thirty-seven lives. Imagine how much more we need to grow and mobilize in order to save animals from all slaughterhouses and factory farms. Apart from working on increasing the number of vegans, we also need to focus more on getting more people involved as activists and leaders. You will definitely not get a law that gives nonhuman animals legal personhood to pass by just increasing the number of vegans in your city. I learned a lot by observing how DxE's San Francisco Bay chapter functioned—giving a lot of importance to building strong and welcoming communities and training members so they could use their skill sets to help grow the movement. Everyone I met had a deep knowledge of nonviolent direct action and how social change happens. But most importantly, I was inspired by the group's ability to dream big and to put their goals into action.

All inspired after the ALC, I started the DxE Pune chapter, and we did several protests, disruptions, trainings, and community-building events. We helped people question social norms that make it okay to eat the dead body of an innocent animal. I realized that justice is not going to be served by itself, that we will have to fight for justice for the animals. Nonviolent direct action is crucial for any movement to succeed.

It's been over three years since I became a part of this movement, and I have grown immensely as a person during this time. The reason this change happened is that I constantly kept unlearning what I had learned. As I went vegan and questioned the notion of eating and using animals, I opened my eyes to other oppressions and injustices in this world and unlearned preconceived notions of what I was expected to do. I have spent all my life in the same city and in a community of people mostly from the same caste and economic class. When that's all you've known, the result is that it narrows your scope, making it harder to accept new ideas or values. You get conditioned by society and have arbitrary ideas of what is right and what is wrong. Your parents, teachers, and friends start shaping and defining your perception of life. That is why children usually have the same political beliefs as their parents. So it's extremely important for us to question some of the traditions that society has conditioned us into believing and to consume new information and knowledge to counter or interrogate things that don't align with our own values or beliefs. For example, the rights women have today were made possible only because someone, somewhere, questioned social norms and dared to think differently. We must be open to learning new ideas and unlearning old ones if we want ourselves and society to grow.

I personally believe there is no inherent purpose to life but it's up to us to *find* purpose in our lives. Having a cause to fight for has made my life so much more meaningful. There is so much cruelty in this world, but we can work to find solutions to most of these problems. We just need individuals to dedicate their lives' purpose to solving them. We need to stop waiting for someone to come and magically create change. What if the person you have been waiting for were actually *you*? I feel like every single person has the power to change the world and reduce suffering if they choose to do so. Upon making such a choice, each individual must find for themselves the best way they can advance their cause.

As for me, I found public activism to be the most direct way to advance the cause of animal liberation; it *is* my moral baseline. I am reminded of this hypothetical situation: Imagine a human is beating a dog on the road. Now, there are three things you can do in this situation. The first thing—and the worst—is to join the human and beat the dog together. The second thing you can do is to choose to not participate and to walk away. I compare this to veganism—nonparticipation in violence. But the third and best thing you can do is to intervene and try to stop the human from beating the dog by whatever means you can think of.

This last option is the one I am compelled to choose, and street activism is my means of helping animals. I feel that it powerfully and effectively brings the issue of animal rights directly into the open: people must acknowledge society's part in the unimaginable violence brought against innocent beings. However, activism can come in all shapes and forms. It doesn't have to be on the streets. One can actively try to dismantle this violent system by—among other things—fundraising, organizing community events, making posters, managing social media, giving speeches, writing books and blogs, promoting plant-based nutrition as a medical professional, bearing witness, or running a vegan business, restaurant, or animal sanctuary. What matters is that you do something that you love and are good at to strengthen the cause. Even if you're not actively involved in advocacy efforts, the ways in which you talk about animal rights and share your story with friends and family can have an impact as well. The important thing is getting people to move in the right direction and motivating them to lead lives of greater compassion.

Since the animal agriculture industry is so powerful, one can lose motivation and hope. In those times, we must remember the sacrifices that past revolutionaries made for us. They fought for us to get the rights that we now enjoy. For example, if the suffragettes had not fought for women's suffrage, then I would never have gotten to experience the freedoms that I have today. If the Indian freedom fighters had not fought British colonial rule, then I wouldn't have gotten to live in a democratic India. Thousands of activists throughout history have sacrificed so much for us to live in the society we live in today. Therefore, I believe it is our duty to use the privilege we have been given to better the world. And to do that, one must have the ability to dream and to believe in one's dreams. My goal is to create a world where all animals have legal personhood. Animals deserve to be safe, happy, and free. I believe my generation has the unique passion to make change happen, but everyone, regardless of their gender, educational background, age, or abilities, can play an important part. There is a social justice warrior in each of us, whom we can choose to embrace.

SARINA FARB
Vegan Educator and Speaker

Sarina Farb is a Midwest-based science educator, speaker, and justice activist with a passion for making the world a better place for all beings. She is the co-founder of the Climate Diet Solution and was co-host of the 2020 Climate Diet Summit. Born in Kansas and raised vegan, Sarina has a lifetime of experience advocating for veganism, climate justice, and sustainable plant-based living. Currently, she serves on the Plant-Based Network advisory committee and is a member of the American Vegan Society Speakers Bureau. Sarina creates empowering and educational content on her website and her YouTube channel, Born Vegan. A former high-school science teacher with a BA in biochemistry and policy studies, she brings critical thinking, nuance, and ethics into conversations about science and sustainability.

MY PARENTS "FORCED" VEGANISM ON ME

As veganism and vegan diets have grown in popularity over the past five years, so has the number of families raising vegan children increased. Unfortunately, veganism is still seen as a radical ideology and diet by much of society. Articles will frequently pop up in the media discussing whether or not vegan parents should even be allowed to "force their values" on their children. A common theme in the articles and commentary is that regardless of their values, parents should let their children choose if they want to be vegan or not. I have even seen people compare veganism to extreme religious brainwashing and cults, making it seem as if any child given a choice in the matter would *obviously* reject veganism. I have also met a number of vegans who have told me that while they have made the personal choice to be vegan, they would never force this on their children, planning instead to let them decide for themselves if they want to go vegan.

As a twenty-six-year-old lifelong vegan whose parents "forced their beliefs" on her as a small child, I have a lot to say on this topic.

The idea that parents shouldn't "force" (a word that really means "educate" in this context) their ethical and moral beliefs on their children is ridiculous, because society itself is not value-neutral. The notion of letting children choose for themselves whether or not they want to be vegan presents a false scenario, in which veganism is viewed as supporting ridiculous and extreme values backed by propaganda. Nonveganism, the default, is thus viewed as neutral and "the norm." Big business, industry, and advertisers create and reinforce this nonvegan norm on a regular basis, which is anything but value-neutral. TV commercials for cheeseburgers, roadside billboards for zoos, and "Got Milk?" ads in magazines and school cafeterias all convey that animals are things and commodities for human use, and that *this* is a value in and of itself.

Similar to when an individual holds a strong moral belief that sexism is wrong and that we shouldn't discriminate against or exploit other humans based on their gender, vegans reject the notion that animals are ours to use and exploit simply because they are of a different species. The same can be said about moral opposition to racism. When the choice between veganism and nonveganism is reframed in this way, it becomes clear that veganism is no more a choice than being against murder, slavery, or any other form of human exploitation.

In the same way that a parent concerned with social justice wouldn't give their children the free choice to be racist or anti-racist, an ethical vegan parent would not offer their child the option of being vegan or not vegan. If vegan parents don't "force" their vegan values and beliefs on their children by teaching and conveying clearly why they are vegan, then society won't hesitate to "force" standard American values on the same children. And without the parents' vegan perspective to counter dominant, mainstream forces, nonveganism may remain unchallenged, with children likely falling prey to the influence and perspectives of industry and big business.

Growing up vegan, I had many of my friends and peers ask things like, "Don't you want to know what cheese tastes like?" or, "Have you ever thought about just sneaking a taste of meat while being away from your parents?" I can honestly say that never once in my life have I been even close to being tempted to taste anything containing animal flesh and secretions. Being on the receiving end of questions like these has often made me feel like I live in a different universe from my peers.

From my very earliest memories, my parents didn't just raise me on a vegan diet. Rather, they laid out a very clear foundation, using age-appropriate reasoning, for what veganism was and why we were vegan. When I was really little, that reasoning was simple, with comments like, "We don't eat animals because it hurts them," and, "We don't drink cow's milk because it's meant for baby cows." As I got older, the explanations got more sophisticated, and conversations about veganism became regular family discussions. We also discussed our duty as citizens of this planet to speak up about injustices and problems of which we were aware. So around seven years of age, with my knowledge of animal exploitation and the environmental havoc that animal agriculture wreaks on the planet, and my family's ideals of speaking out against injustice, I felt compelled to share the truth with my friends and peers. Although I won't say I was the most tactful or effective at the time, I did my best to speak out against the atrocities I saw. This practice of repeatedly speaking out on issues of justice set the tone for all of my actions and choices since then.

To have been raised vegan is the biggest blessing I could have ever asked for. Not only has it given me peace of mind, knowing that I have never intentionally participated in harming animals, but it has also taught me to view the entire world in a different light and to think critically about everything. By seeing past the propaganda that backs and spreads the pervasive belief in society that it's okay to use animals, I've learned to turn a more critical eye to everything that society presents as normal and to never take anything at face value. So what do I, as someone who had veganism "forced" on her, think about parents forcing veganism on their children? They are no different from parents who "force" anti-racist or anti-sexist beliefs and values on their children.

GWENNA HUNTER

Heart Activist and Storyteller

Gwenna Hunter is the creator of Vegans of LA, Vegans for Black Lives Matter, and Health Campaign. She also manages several Vegan Food Aid programs for Vegan Outreach, working with organizations such as Black Women for Wellness, Black Lives Matter LA, Black Women Farmers of LA, and the LGBT Center South. In addition, Gwenna is involved with the Animal Save Movement; she manages the Mutual Food Aid program, working with the Downtown Crenshaw Coalition, and the Los Angeles Health Save Campaign. Gwenna has resided in Los Angeles since July 4, 2014, having previously lived in Cleveland, Miami, Charlotte, Texas, and Atlanta.

THE POWER OF ISIS

I was in the fourth or fifth grade and coming home from school. I could tell something was off. The energy felt strange to me. I was told by my stepfather to take out a white bag of trash to the garbage. It was odd to me because the trash bag wasn't full and it felt like something heavy was inside. But he was not one to be questioned by a child, so I did as I was told. After coming back inside, I wondered where Isis was. He was an all-Black, shiny, beautiful cat with glowy, magical eyes; he loved me, and I loved him. Once, he got stuck up in the ceiling area in the basement, and he wouldn't trust anyone to help him down except for me. We had a bond that I knew was special. It was my first experience that I remember of loving an animal. My stepfather was medically diagnosed with paranoid schizophrenia. Medications barely kept his episodes under control, but when he was motivated by his own jealous feelings and competitiveness, his illness would often bring out the worst in him, which would usually lead to violence and verbal abuse toward me.

It wasn't long after taking out the white trash bag that I was told by him, with a smirk on his face that also indicated some ill form of satisfaction, that the trash I had taken out contained my Isis. Apparently, Isis and my stepfather had had a confrontation, and my stepfather had decided to take the life of my Isis. I was devastated. My little heart was completely broken over this news. My beloved Isis lay slumped inside of a plastic bag inside of a trash can. Where was his little soul? Had he suffered? Had he hoped that I would return home and rescue him? Where was that part of him that loved me? Had it died, too, or was it somewhere hiding, waiting for me to find it? I wanted to know. This experience changed me in such a way that I became fearful of cats for a period of time in my life. I would be an adult in my late mid-thirties before I would give myself permission to connect with a cat again.

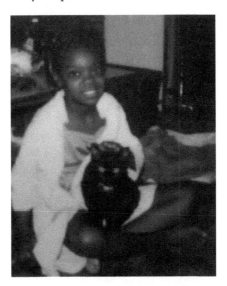

When I became vegan in 2016, I began soaking up all of the information that I had never been taught regarding protein, factory farming, dairy, etc. I also began learning about cultures that consume dogs and cats. I couldn't believe it. My cat companion Chyna was so full of life and love. She was love and affection wrapped in fur. How could anyone look at her and become hungry? I could not imagine. But then again, in our American culture, we see chickens, pigs, cows, turkeys, sea animals, even baby lambs as sources of food. These animals love their mamas and their mamas love them. The powers that be have done a masterful job on the human civilization. They have convinced the majority of us that these precious beings belong to us to do as we please. Sound familiar? Our species has even manipulated holy scriptures to drive this message even further.

* * *

When I was around twenty-three years of age, I began having really abnormal symptoms. I would have cold sweats and extreme pain in my lower back and abdomen—pain so bad that I would often pass out. My symptoms included nausea and frequent vomiting. I would often end up in the emergency room, each time with a misdiagnosis. At first, I was told I had an ulcer and was prescribed medication. That didn't work. Then they decided to diagnose me with kidney stones. That wasn't it either. Perplexed as to why these symptoms would randomly appear, I began thinking about what I was doing or eating each time an episode occurred. The only common denominator was that prior to each of these episodes, I had consumed cows. I realized that my body no longer wanted cows inside of it. And if I decided to ignore the message, my body would turn on me and remind me of it. Once I eliminated cows from my diet, the painful attacks ended. It would be just a few months more until I decided to also stop consuming pigs. Both of these decisions had nothing to do with the actual animals and everything to do with self-preservation.

Fast forward to the year 2008, when I was asked to do the Daniel Fast by a religious friend. Here is what Wikipedia says about the Daniel Fast: *The Daniel Fast is a religious partial fast that is popular among Evangelical Protestants in North America in which meat, wine, and other rich foods are avoided in favor of vegetables and water for typically three weeks in order to be more sensitive to God. The fast is based on the lifelong kosher diet of the Jewish hero Daniel in the Biblical Book of Daniel and the three-week mourning fast in which Daniel abstained from all meat and wine.* She was basically asking me to go vegan for twenty-eight days. The purpose of doing the Daniel Fast, for me, was to have a more powerful ability to manifest. I agreed.

This decision would lead me on the path to veganism. I consumed a lot of potatoes to keep myself full. I remember feeling lighter and happier. When it was time for my moon cycle to visit, I had no cramps, no discomfort, no acne breakouts, and my emotions were well balanced. At the end of the twenty-eight days, I decided I would reimplement dairy (because I needed my calcium!) and began living a vegetarian lifestyle.

I remember one day having a waking supernatural experience. My mom was eating a chicken meal from a fast food restaurant. All of a sudden, I heard a high-pitched sound in both ears. Everything felt like it'd stopped. I was engulfed in what felt like surround sound. I could hear my mom chewing the food, as if someone had turned the volume up to ten times the level I was used to hearing. My sense of smell was magnified to a superhuman level. The chicken smelled rotten. The sound of the chewing turned my stomach because, all of a sudden, I understood (temporarily) that it was the sound of a dead body being consumed. The entire experience may have lasted fewer than thirty seconds. At the time, I didn't understand why this was happening to me, and I wouldn't understand until several years later.

My vegetarian journey would continue for another eight years while I resided mostly in North Carolina and for a spell in Dallas, Texas. I was transitioning in my career and decided to visit Los Angeles, California, for a few weeks. During my stay, I decided to give LA a chance and make it permanent. After a couple of months, things took a turn for bad, and I found myself on the verge of being completely houseless with my cat. I could not afford the typical LA rent but ended up encountering someone online who would be my Angel for a time. Her name is Rhea Roma. She allowed me and my Chyna to rent her couch. When I visited her eclectic home, there were other cats and dogs running around. One of the first things she told me was that she was a vegan and that I could not bring meat or dairy products into her home. I let her know that I was a vegetarian and that I was more than willing to forgo bringing dairy into her home, so she didn't have to worry.

I remember one day seeing Rhea in a very sad mood, crying. She said, "I can't bear to think about what they are doing to the animals right now!" She was balled up in a knot. In my mind, not having yet made the connection, I couldn't connect to what she was saying, nor did I understand her emotions, which seemed quite extreme and exaggerated to me at the time. Little did I know that I myself would have many of the same moments in the future. Every so often, Rhea would give me a lecture about dairy products, but again I would think she was being extreme. After a couple of months, I was able to graduate from renting a couch to renting a room in a shared apartment. It was there that I would end up having a supernatural dream that would change the path of my life forever.

I dreamed that I was flying in the sky, overlooking a beautiful bright green pasture. I noticed a beautiful cow looking up at me. Our eyes connected and when they did, it was like I had flown inside of this cow and become one with her. I *was* the cow. We merged and I felt her sorrow, her grief, her love, her excitement, and her joy as she gave birth to her children, loved her children, loved and enjoyed the companionship of humans. I emerged from the dream in shock, knowing what I had experienced had to be real, but of course, I questioned it. I was crying uncontrollably because what I felt more than anything was animals' immense capacity to love. It was a love that was pure and kind and gentle and sweet. It was unconditional. But how could a cow be capable of this? After all, weren't cows put here for us? As I cried and sat up in my bed, I suddenly felt a physical warmth on my chest—right where my heart resided. I took my right hand and put it on the warm spot, and I was paralyzed by the most beautiful feeling of tranquility and complete peace. It was so warm and loving and soft. It felt so good that I could have died from the experience. I knew that what I was experiencing wasn't my imagination but the cow giving me a piece of her heart and letting me know that those like her love, too, and that they love us.

It would be a few weeks later that I would come across the video by Erin Janus called "Dairy Is F-cking Scary," from which I would see for myself what these cows go through. As a woman, I identified their experience as rape and as a Black woman, I easily saw that they are enslaved by humanity, the majority of which does not have a clue that this is going on. I felt I needed to shout from the mountaintops to wake up everyone I knew would listen. I soon realized it's not that easy to wake people up. I knew that I was destined to work in the movement. It was the first time in my life that I was a part of something this big and that I had this much desire to help wake up humanity.

The Council of Pigs

I had another experience that was also beyond the normal limits of reality. I found myself in a different space and time as I was standing outside of a slaughterhouse where there were cows and pigs standing in line, waiting for their turn to be slaughtered. I instantly had a telepathic connection with them, and I knew that they had full awareness of what was going to happen. I began crying and yelling at them, telling them not to reincarnate back onto this planet and not to come back to Earth because we keep killing and hurting their kind. All of a sudden, one of the pigs turned to me and spoke to me in the most powerful male voice, saying: "We will keep coming back again and again until you all get it right. We love you all that much. Our suffering gives some of your lives purpose." He then sent an impulse of his love to my heart and it was so incredibly pure and beautiful. This impulse let me know that it's not just that we're trying to save them—they are also saving us.

I often think of my Isis. He has even visited my dreams, letting me know that his time being cut short wasn't anyone's fault and that part of his experience had been to take some of the violence that might have been meant for me. Isis was my first animal love. I do this work in honor of him—and all animals and humans. We are all born sovereign. Rights are not to be taken or given. You are here to stand in your power. You are the solution. You are the bringer of light. You are the good news. Even though it may feel like this world hurts you at times, you must remember to be joy. Love always. Laugh as much as you can. Cry when you need to. Call on a friend or loved one when you are angry and in pain. One of the most powerful forms you can take on is that of an activist. You can help activate and awaken people's hearts and transform their minds away from the programming of this illusion. You were born for this. We are Activists and are here to help transform and heal the world and restore heaven on Earth. We may fuss and fight, but we cannot do this work without love. Remember who you are and why you are here. Let's create a new world together.

SANDRA ISOBEL KYLE

The Singing Vegan

A vegan since 2010, Sandra Isobel Kyle lives in Whanganui, New Zealand, and has been a writer and activist for animal rights since the 1990s. Her book *Glass Walls* and her website endanimalslaughter.org call for all slaughterhouses in New Zealand to close by 2025. Sandra produced the animal rights radio show *Safe and Sound* for four and a half years. She is one of two country liaisons for the Save Movement in New Zealand; a short film, *2025*, was made about her solitary slaughterhouse vigils. In 2018, Sandra received the Philip Wollen Animal Welfare Award. Dubbed by the mainstream media as "The Singing Vegan," she was nominated in 2021 for the Assisi Award, named after the patron saint of animals, St. Francis of Assisi.

A MOMENTOUS TIME TO BE LIVING THROUGH

But if you go again and again to the waters, there–under the wheeling of skylark, under the wings of blue heron, under the brightness of duck wing, in the shallows where small fish dart, under the willows where the pool is deep and lucid, around the next bend where the light falls so hard on the ripples it splinters and bounces like rain–there you might find your answers.—Jillian Sullivan[1]

Restless and Seeking

I grew up in the 1950s in a new state housing suburb on the outskirts of Auckland, formerly a wilderness of swamps, streams, quarries, and scrubland. Family life was often fraught, and when I wanted to escape, I would seek out a couple of "happy places" within walking distance from our house. One was a stagnant pond near a culvert on the main road leading to town. The other was a stream that flowed behind blackberry bushes on land still untouched by suburban spread; black eels swam in this weed-tangled waterway, just as their ancestors had done since the early Miocene. At the algae-covered pond, I would crouch on my heels to watch the teeming activity. In those days, when human activity had impacted Nature less, the ribbitting of frogs was a signature sound in our neighbourhood after dark.

I loved to ride my bike to the large hill the suburb was named after, Mount Roskill, and flop on my back in the grass, looking for faces of people and animals in the clouds. Even now, in my seventies, I still find comfort in gazing up at the very large and down at the very small: down at scarabs tunneling dung into the earth—a four-million-year-old solution for enriching our soils; up at the horizon's thin line; down at blind tubular earthworms turning over the turf; and up at faint grey smudges in the night sky that are really blazing suns in distant galaxies.

I adored our family cats and dogs and made a fuss over every animal I saw. Our small garden shed became a surgery where I looked after stunned or injured birds. In short, I have felt a deep connection with other forms of life and a fascination with Nature from an early age, and even considered becoming a nature writer like my friend Jillian. Yet as diverse and beautiful as Nature is, it is also devastatingly brutal. Hunger, thirst, disease, conflict, fear, and psychological stress are the lot of other animals, as is premature death. There are endless examples of this, such as turtle hatchlings who, left by their mothers to fend for themselves, struggle on their little legs to cross the sand to the relative safety of the sea. Within moments of hatching, the vast majority are picked off by crabs and seagulls. To me, each one of these babies is a precious individual; to Nature, they're a cold statistic to ensure the survival of the fittest. As circumstances did not arrange themselves for me to become a writer, I instead became a teacher—of office systems, of all things, and then English as a Second Language. But my sensitivity to life around me, my quest to find meaning, and my love for our fellow creatures were there from early on.

I left home while still a teenager, traveled, encountered hardships, and became a spiritual seeker. I began to understand that the world we had created was a symptom of our own consciousness and that the only real way to solve our problems was to grow spiritually, to evolve. Becoming vegetarian was part of that for me. I had already given up meat and fish after reading Peter Singer's *Animal Liberation*, a seminal book for activists of my generation. I remember lying in my bed, reading about the horrors of factory farming, my hands shaking as I turned the pages. More than forty-five years later, I can still recall photos of little veal calves being tethered and kept in darkness their entire lives in order to produce the tender, pale flesh coveted by meat eaters. In the industry, baby calves are sometimes so crippled that they have to be helped onto the truck that carries them, at just eighteen weeks old, to the slaughter plant. I was deeply shocked that humans could be so cruel, but there was still a lot I didn't piece together. This all changed ten years ago when I learned of the fate of unwanted, mainly male "bobby" calves sent to slaughter at four days old, and I went vegan overnight. It was also the watershed for my embarking on serious activism for animals.

A couple of years later, having reached sixty-five and been guaranteed a pension from the government, I was able to retire from my job and throw myself into animal rights. Today, I work from a number of different platforms, but dearest to my heart are the slaughterhouse vigils I do as part of the Animal Save Movement. Founder Anita Krajnc based her inspiration on this premise attributed to Tolstoy, "When the suffering of another creature causes you to feel pain, do not submit to the initial desire to flee from the suffering one, but on the contrary, come closer, as close as you can to him who suffers, and try to help him."[2] And seeking to assuage suffering has always been my inclination. It is true we can do nothing about Nature's cruelty, but we cannot blame Nature for the institutional and systemic domination and oppression of animals. This is humanity's crime, and therefore, it is possible for us to do something about it.

"The Singing Vegan"

A few years ago, I was driving in the countryside when I passed a stock car filled with sheep. The driver was off collecting more animals, so I had the opportunity to spend time with them. It was heartbreaking for me to see these gentle creatures, much more intelligent and complex than they're reputed to be,[3] and as I stroked them, I had the idea of singing to them the way a mother would sing a lullaby to her child. I had visited India many times and lived in ashrams, and a mantra came to my mind. I videoed it and put it on social media, and when the press heard about it, they dubbed me "The Singing Vegan."

In the town I am currently living in, there are two slaughterhouses, which I visit once or twice a week, often by myself. One is for sheep, lambs, and bobby calves, the other for cows and pigs. If I'm lucky, the truck arriving at the sheep and bobby slaughterhouse has to stop at the gates to let another vehicle out, and I can have a few moments with the animals. The frightened, bewildered eyes of the babies relax a little as I stroke their noses and ears, speak softly, play music, or sing to them before they are taken onto the premises and out of sight. The cow and pig slaughterhouse is on a main thoroughfare, and it is possible to have a good view of the animals arriving and being unloaded into holding pens. Anyone who has heard a pig cry knows how bloodcurdling the sound is—something between a scream and a roar.

The air at this particular slaughterhouse is filled with loud noises—passing traffic, whirring machinery, metal doors, and truck compartments slamming open and shut, as well as the "hup hups" of human voices goading frightened animals to move. Intelligent, aware pigs cower in the corners of the truck, as workers wave sticks with plastic bags in front of their eyes. As soon as they are locked inside their pens, they begin to scream, triggering the cows next door, who bellow and moo plaintively. Standing on my stepladder, I get a good view into the cows' pens, and much is revealed. Their behaviors—mooing, stamping, eye rolling, slumping, head hanging, restlessness—show that they are stressed and depressed and that inside their body vehicles, so superficially different from our own, they are emotional, sentient beings with the same capacity as our own to feel joy, fear, and pain, and with the same desire not to be killed. I recognize in them the identical mysterious life energy that is in all creation and that has fascinated me since I was a child. Along with thousands of others in the Save Movement who bear witness to and document these animals' lives, I want the world to see what I see. When I look at a calf, a cow, a sheep, a pig at the slaughterhouse, I don't see just a body—I feel a being; I see a soul.

Evolving to a Higher Consciousness

It has now been five years that I have been doing my vigils, and it doesn't get any easier. I can still scarcely believe what I witness with my own eyes. Can this really be happening? How can we still be doing this to sentient beings in 2020?

Sometimes, it's the little "epiphanies" that hurt the most. At the cow slaughterhouse, there is a fountain attached to the iron bars on the side of the pens. As I watch the animals lower their massive heads to suck up the water, I feel deep sorrow, which doesn't seem to make any sense. Why should watching them drink make me so sad?

I think there are a number of reasons for this. Cows are similar to us. We share the same evolutionary development and belong to the same class of mammals. Like us, they have a four-chambered heart, specialized teeth, three middle-ear bones, and a neocortex region in the brain. Like us, they are complex, possess intelligence and awareness, and form attachments to their families and friends. They are our kin, but instead of loving and respecting them, we treat them like commodities. We line them up to slit their throats because we want to eat them.

Our abusive Master–Subject relationship with the animals we raise for food is mind-numbing in its scope—up to seventy billion land animals killed every year, trillions when you factor in sea life. Cows are larger than us—700 kilograms is the average weight of a slaughter steer in New Zealand—but we are much more intelligent and powerful. We exploit their vulnerability, even foster their trust and then betray them. No, we are not just their masters, we are their very creators. We bring them into the world to satisfy our own desires by taking away their own.

As I stand and watch, I can sense the cows' desperate psychological state. They are anxious, fearful, depressed, confused. They try to understand what is happening, but it is new, they can't make it out. They smell blood and know something is very wrong; I understand that there is an element of displacement behavior in their drinking. Knowing I cannot save them is the worst feeling, but what I can do, I do. I comfort them, talk to them, sing to them, document their lives, and share all of this on social media.

In my senior years, I can see how the strands of my life are coming together. An insight I had early on in the development of our movement was that the vegan revolution is an essential part of the evolution of consciousness that humanity has to undergo in order to solve our problems. It is the first step in creating a nonviolent world. Aided by, among other things, the Internet and rising plant-based protein technologies, just as mountains are eroded by constant wind and precipitation, a tiny minority of animal activists are breaking the iron chains of habit and tradition to create a better, brighter future for all Earthlings. I can clearly see that the world is turning away from the violence of killing animals for food, just as it rejected human slavery in the nineteenth century and gave women the vote in the early twentieth. The repercussions of this change will be transformational. I feel humbled and give thanks that I and my fellow animal activists have a part to play in this momentous point in history that we are living through.

CLAUDIA LIFTON

Denver Director and Festival Outreach Coordinator,
Factory Farming Awareness Coalition

Claudia Lifton has been with the Factory Farming Awareness Coalition since 2015. Prior to working with FFAC, she traveled throughout Africa and Southeast Asia, working with locals to address concerns ranging from poaching, shark finning, overfishing, water access, animal tourism exploitation, to wildlife trafficking. She spent three summers working at Catskill Animal Sanctuary in New York, helping to run Camp Kindness, a summer camp where children learned about farmed animals, plant-based diet and nutrition, and effective advocacy. In her free time, Claudia enjoys attending concerts and festivals, hiking, camping, and cuddling with rescued farmed animals at her favorite sanctuaries.

STORIES OF A "BUG GIRL"

It started with earthworms. While other kids played with Barbie dolls and Tonka trucks, I played with annelids and insects. I quickly became Highmount Avenue's resident animal rescuer. Neighbors would call my mom if they found injured butterflies, baby birds, or snakes. As my rescue services became better known, we had to convert our downstairs bathroom into a makeshift rehabilitation center, filled with creatures in need of a helping hand. The derogatory nickname I was given by my classmates in elementary school (which I later reclaimed as a badge of honor) was "Bug Girl." While other kids played on the swings during recess, I would take the caterpillars I had brought to school in the little carrier I wore around my neck for walks around the schoolyard. There were times when I ran to the principal's office in tears after I had seen schoolmates use sunlight and their magnifying glasses to kill bugs on the playground. I was incensed and confused by the cruelty they inflicted on these innocent little creatures.

During my first year of college, I started to think critically about the many ways in which animals are exploited. I realized that loving animals wasn't enough, so I started volunteering at Paws Across Oswego County (PAOC). Marjorie and Ed, who ran the shelter, taught me what it meant to devote one's life to saving animals. Watching their love and devotion transform traumatized dogs into trusting individuals taught me selflessness and patience. They also taught me that instead of merely treating wounds, we could prevent them. I began assisting with their community outreach, going into schools and community centers to encourage adopting animals rather than buying from pet stores.

After graduating, I read about a contest, sponsored by Global Vision International (GVI), that seemed tailor-made for me. I was chosen out of 5000 applicants to spend all of 2013 blogging for GVI about my time volunteering in five countries at twelve of their research and conservation sites. In Kenya, Thailand, Mexico, and South Africa, I worked with rescued and injured wildlife. Through research initiatives, we educated local communities and governments about the dangers of shark finning, overfishing, and wildlife poaching. But it was during my time off that my determination to rescue animals truly developed.

In Nadi, Fiji, I spent my free time volunteering at a local animal shelter, and using the connections I'd built with the local community, I started the first-ever spay and neuter clinic on a small island of Fiji. While in Thailand, I spent my days off leafleting outside of elephant-riding camps and tiger-tourism centers, educating tourists about the violent, exploitative nature of the wildlife tourism and trafficking industries. Working directly with elephants, cheetahs, baboons, and other rescued wild animals was life-affirming, but I was—and am—continuously drawn toward advocacy and education—preventing the abuse that leads to these animals having to be rescued in the first place.

While taking a short trip to Laos to renew my Thai visa, I met a terrified, malnourished baby macaque chained to a pole outside of a mechanic shop. I knew right away that I couldn't leave him there to suffer. After many hours of begging and bargaining, I was able to persuade his captors to let me take him to a vet and bring him back the next day. Of course, I had no intention of returning little Hug (short for Nahuglai, "forever loved" in Laotian), so we set off on a five-day adventure, traveling together via bus and boat, making our way to the sanctuary where he now lives with an adopted family of his own kind.

Rescuing Hug was incredibly rewarding, but it was also time-consuming and exhausting. It helped me realize that I couldn't just save animals one by one. So when I returned to the US, I knew my life's work would be devoted to ending the largest system of animal abuse—factory farming.

I next worked at Catskill Animal Sanctuary (CAS), a farmed animal rescue in upstate New York. At CAS, I helped develop the curriculum for and run a summer camp (Camp Kindness) that was created to inspire and educate children to become animal advocates and stewards of the earth. Many of the kids who attended Camp Kindness had never met a pig, cow, or chicken. They quickly fell in love with the animals they'd once seen only as body parts on their dinner plates.

One of those kids, whom I'll call Ian, asked if we could have bacon for lunch on the first day of camp and commented about how "delicious" the resident pigs looked. (Much of my story as an animal rights activist can be summarized by variations of the phrase, "Mmm . . . bacon," as I'm sure many vegans can relate to.) I used his comments as an opportunity to talk about how intelligent and wonderful pigs are and made sure that Ian spent plenty of time with them throughout the week. For his first encounter with the pigs, Ian was given a handful of pumpkin seeds. Wonder replaced mockery as he edged his hand closer to Jasmine's inquisitive snout. Ian laughed as Jasmine ate out of his palm, and within moments, he was close enough to kiss her. Ian fell in love with these gentle, sensitive creatures as quickly as I had. By the third day of camp, Ian was writing angry letters to Smithfield, condemning its mistreatment of pigs, and making decorative flyers about the wonders of pigs to pass around his neighborhood. By the end of the week, Ian had become a most ardent vegan activist.

My experience at CAS was my first time working directly with and for farmed animals. Getting to intimately know animals who had been raised for food and rescued from slaughter turned an abstract concept I'd had into reality. This deeper understanding knocked the wind out of me. As happens to many newly minted animal advocates, I fell into a depression. The enormity of the institutionalized violence against animals led me to feelings of helplessness and hopelessness. It was then that I met Katie Cantrell. Katie founded the Factory Farming Awareness Coalition, where I've worked since 2015. Katie taught me how to communicate the vegan message without alienating others. She gave me the tools to turn difficult conversations into transformational ones and taught me how to channel my pain and anger into action. It was during my time learning from Katie that the darkness lifted.

My job at FFAC is to inspire and empower people to create a more just, compassionate, and sustainable food system. I speak to middle school, high school, and college students about the impacts of factory farming on the earth and its inhabitants. It is empowering to know that as I foster empathy and awareness in young people, I can help create a world in which fewer animals will suffer at the hands of humans.

I also moved away from single-issue advocacy and toward a holistic approach. As a presenter, I meet people where they are. If they are concerned about their health, I talk to them about the ways in which the standard American diet promotes disease. If a professor is teaching a class on environmental ethics, I present data on the water, land, and carbon footprint of meat, dairy, and egg production. For those fighting for human rights, I address the prevalence of environmental racism, workers' rights abuses, and community destruction caused by industrial animal agriculture. Everyone cares about something, and I tap into people's passions to drive them into action.

This work is deeply fulfilling and worthwhile. It is also frustrating and emotionally draining. The presentations I give to thousands of young people each year are provoking to many of the attendees, as I am challenging assumptions these students have held since birth. Inevitably, many of them become defensive. While speaking to a school assembly of six hundred high-school juniors, I saw two girls dressed in bacon costumes in the front row. After the presentation had ended, I noticed them waiting for me by the stage. With guilty smiles, they told me they would be retiring their bacon costumes for good and wanted to change their eating habits as a result of what I had taught them.

Around that time, another opportunity arose. Live music and festivals have been my haven for as long as I can remember; the joy and abandon I feel while dancing under the stars to my favorite bands provide me with the energy and healing I need to continue being the best animal advocate I can be. However, after going vegan, I found myself frustrated by the contradiction in these purportedly hyper-spiritual environmentalists, who were preaching about the importance of kindness and compassion while simultaneously contributing to the largest ethical and environmental catastrophe in human history by consuming factory-farmed meat.

If I wanted to impact this group of people involved in a scene that meant so much to me, I knew I would have to create a tailored outreach strategy. I asked several musician friends in the transformational music festival scene to send me quotes about their reasons for going vegan, and I created promotional materials targeted at this segment of festival goers. In 2016, I started vending at music festivals across the country with virtual reality headsets from Animal Equality that show life through the eyes of animals raised for food.

As it always seems to do, my story brings us back, once again, to bacon. While vending at a festival in Pennsylvania, I saw a young man walking by our booth wearing a bacon costume. After being offered a $10 bribe, he was persuaded to see through the eyes of a pig—from life to death—via virtual reality. With tears in his eyes, he immediately removed his costume and pledged to never consume pig flesh again. A year later, I ran into him while vending at the same festival, and he proudly announced that he had gone vegan. These experiences continue to remind me that even a man dressed as bacon isn't out of reach.

I've come a long way from "Bug Girl." I still love all creatures, big and small, but I've moved on from spending my days playing with earthworms and spiders to advocating for cows and pigs, from preaching to my fellow nine-year-olds about the cruelty of killing ants to standing in front of thousands of students a year, entreating them to stop harming chickens and turkeys. I've moved on from battling my teachers when they'd try to make us dissect frogs in the classroom to battling one of the most powerful industries on Earth, determined to intimidate me and my fellow activists into silence. I know that together, we will never stop fighting until every cage is empty.

JAMES O'TOOLE

Co-director of Communications, Animal Save Movement

James O'Toole became vegan in 2010 after reading about the horrors of the dairy industry, and an activist in 2014 after bearing witness at a Save vigil. Connecting with a cow arriving for slaughter was for him a transformational event, and animal rights became a priority in his life. James immediately began volunteering with Toronto Pig Save, and activism soon became his full-time focus. Previously, James worked in the finance industry as a stockbroker and wrote market commentary articles for a newspaper. He is also a certified personal trainer and nutritionist.

IS THIS SOMETHING YOU WANT TO SUPPORT?

When the suffering of another creature causes you to feel pain, do not submit to the initial desire to flee from the suffering one, but on the contrary, come closer, as close as you can to him who suffers, and try to help him.—Leo Tolstoy[4]

Bearing witness to suffering nonhuman animals is a duty we all share, just as helping humans in need is a duty we all share. It is innate in humans to help those who are suffering. But animal agriculture has successfully hidden its victims from public view, and has, through clever marketing and advertising, hoodwinked consumers so much that they no longer realize what they are contributing to and what they are supporting. Animal rights activists try to reveal the truth to the public through many forms of activism: street outreach and leafleting, virtual reality outreach, undercover filming of the insides of slaughterhouses, and Cubes of Truth, whereby passersby in busy public places see and hopefully are moved by images of the horrors of animal agriculture displayed on screens. I have participated in all of these forms of activism, but nothing, in my opinion, is as instantly transformative and effective as bearing witness.

Bearing witness is in many ways a simple act that anyone can do. At Animal Save vigils, people gather outside slaughterhouses (or other sites of animal exploitation) and wait for the transport trucks containing animals to arrive. These trucks usually come from factory farms, where pigs, cows, chickens, or other animals have been bred and raised in hellish conditions, often never having seen sunlight until the trip to the slaughterhouse. The animals are usually still babies. Most animals killed for human consumption are still in their infancy—a few weeks old in the case of chickens, a few months old for pigs, and a year and a half old for cows. It doesn't make economic sense for them to live any longer than that. Of course, in the eyes of animal agriculture, they are simply products to be sold. It is not financially expedient to let these sentient beings live one day longer than is absolutely necessary. So they are sent to slaughter. If activists aren't waiting for the animals outside the slaughterhouse to document their plight and give them a moment of compassion, a drink of water, then no one is. They live their entire short lives unacknowledged, from birth to violent death.

Vigils are always traumatic. I see no differences that matter between a dog and a pig. If you imagine how you would feel bearing witness to a truck full of dogs arriving for slaughter, dehydrated and terrified, then you may have an understanding of how difficult I and other activists find animal vigils. Something that helps with the trauma is the growing supportive community of people all refusing to look away any longer. As soon as I joined Toronto Cow Save and started posting the images daily on social media, it helped me deal with the trauma to know I was shining a light on what the industry wants to hide—that these animals are individuals who do not want to die. Vegans are living proof that we do not need to kill them to be healthy, to live.

When we meet the victims of animal agriculture, we see them not as commodities or objects or "food," but as individuals who want to live. We see their terror, fear, hopelessness, confusion; we see their pain and suffering. We realize that if it were our own animal companions, our dogs or cats, in the trucks, the emotions would be the same. We realize that if we ourselves were in the trucks, the emotions would be the same. It is impossible not to be moved by the experience.

As a result of this new awareness, the thought of continuing to consume animal flesh becomes abhorrent to those not yet vegan. Even for established vegans such as myself, bearing witness for the first time makes it impossible *not* to fight for them, the victims. It is truly a transformational experience. Fighting for animal rights becomes a priority. Speaking up for the victims becomes a priority. It is not that they are voiceless, as anyone who has borne witness can testify. They are extremely vocal, as is evident in their desperate pleas for help, their screams of terror, but they are the exploited, who simply do not have the means to stop their oppression. They need us to advocate on their behalf.

In society, we are conditioned from infancy to believe the lies that it is normal, natural, and necessary to consume animal products. It is up to those of us who have broken the disconnect to inform the public that these myths are not true and that believing them is not only wrong but incredibly destructive to our planet, our health, and of course, the billions of animals who are abused, tortured, and murdered at the hands of humans every single year. Bearing witness allows activists to do this in the most visceral and raw way possible. The footage captured forces the public to confront and acknowledge the reality of their choices. The animals who are consumed are not simply products on a shelf, with no more history than a tin of beans; they are the carved-up body parts of individuals who wanted to live, who had families, and who felt pain and grief.

By extension, bearing witness challenges the public's apathy and demands that if people are appalled at this injustice and have a heart full of sorrow and empathy for these animals, then they are left with one inconvenient, unpleasant, yet undeniable fact: if they are not vegan, they are paying for this to happen.

Without the demand, billions of land animals and trillions of marine animals around the world would not be killed every year.

Bearing witness brings these individuals momentarily "back to life"; it forces people to question their beliefs and their conditioning and ask themselves—is this really something they want to support?

CURTIS VOLLMAR

Animal Liberation Activist

Curtis Vollmar has been active for the animals since 2017. He is most proud of his work with Direct Action Everywhere (DxE) that exposed and successfully shut down Iowa Select Farms's use of ventilation shutdown (VSD). The VSD story was uncovered by Pulitzer Prize–winning journalist Glenn Greenwald. In college, Curtis was a D1 All-American track athlete with a 4:06 mile to his name, and he continues to train to this day. Outside of activism, he enjoys any form of competition, from video games, yard games, to *Magic: The Gathering.* He also appreciates a great-fitting pair of skinny jeans.

GET INVOLVED

From Bacon, Lettuce, and Tomato to Jail

On a Tuesday night in November of 2017, I was hosting a social gathering for a dozen friends. Such nights were for conversation, music, beer, and board games. The main attraction was the food, and that night, BLTs were on the menu. My job was to get artisan bacon from a local butcher shop.

Right when my friends were scheduled to be over, I was scrolling through YouTube, looking for a music playlist, and a video started autoplaying as if it were an advertisement. Its title: "Gary Yourofsky— The Best Speech You Will Ever Hear." I was curious, and I clicked.

Five minutes later, people started to arrive, and I got up to play host. We all had a great time sharing stories and playing the game *Settlers of Catan*, but I couldn't get my mind off of the speech. As soon as everyone had left, I immediately resumed watching. My attention was rapt; the language Yourofsky used and the manner in which he spoke were captivating. The video ended at around 1:00 a.m., and I fell asleep shortly thereafter.

The next morning, I threw out all the animal products in my fridge and cupboards. One month later, I wrote an email about activism that resulted in my being fired from my job. Two months later, I started disrupting grocery stores and restaurants to speak up for animals. Three months later, I was arrested at a mass protest at a slaughterhouse in Tar Heel, North Carolina. Four months later, I started organizing small-scale protests and demonstrations.

My name is Curtis Vollmar, and I have been an animal rights activist since that November 2017 edition of "BLT night."

Who Are Activists? Where Do They Come From?

Eve Ensler, American playwright and feminist activist best known for her play *The Vagina Monologues,* had this to say:

> An activist is someone who cannot help but fight for something. That person is not usually motivated by a need for power or money or fame, but in fact is driven slightly mad by some injustice, some cruelty, some unfairness, so much so that he or she is compelled by some internal moral engine to act to make it better.[5]

This excerpt deeply resonates with me. Once you've seen the footage from the slaughterhouses, once you've gone into the farms and heard the animals' cries, there is no turning back. Once you've learned about the scale, horror, and violence of and secrecy surrounding the practices in modern animal agriculture, there is no turning back. The world doesn't seem to be what it was before, and you *need* to make it better. You're now driven mad. What is this "internal moral engine"? Is it only activists who have it? I don't believe this to be true. I believe all humans know right from wrong. I believe that empathy is innate and violence is learned. The problem is that we've been conditioned by society to not only suppress our innate and deepest sense of empathy, but also shun and ridicule those who openly display it. From the moment we're born, we're inundated with TV commercials, billboards, and other advertisements telling us animals are commodities.

Items such as McDonald's "Happy Meals" specifically target children and perpetuate the false and violent ideology that animals exist for humans to use and exploit. This narrative, known as speciesism, is reinforced by social and cultural norms, our friends and families, and even religious institutions. Speciesism is so deeply rooted in society that we never even consider the animals, let alone see them as victims. Unlearning speciesism is the first step in harnessing the power of your "internal moral engine."

So who become activists? Where do they come from? The simple answer is: anyone, from anywhere. Having been involved in activism for a few years now, I can say that the animal rights community is one of the most diverse communities I've ever been in. I've met and become friends with people from all walks of life: gay and straight, young and old, rich and poor, black and white, foreign and domestic, able-bodied and disabled, and so on. This speaks to the power of the message. Nonviolence and empathy for all sentient beings are universal truths that speak to all those brave enough to accept them.

What Can I Do?

After I was introduced to animal rights and the notion of speciesism, I began to challenge myself and the world around me. I quickly adopted a plant-based diet and swore off any consumer products that were not animal-friendly. The corporate establishment I was working for at the time was challenged by the activism materials I brought into the workspace. I began going to larger protests and started organizing demonstrations. I was also involved with a political campaign to get a friend and fellow animal rights activist elected mayor. All of these actions, though they have a common goal, use different tactics and can be categorized under different Theories of Change.

Paul Engler, activist, educator, and author of *This Is an Uprising*, has classified five different Theories of Change, which entail, respectively, personal transformation, alternatives, inside game, structure organizing, and mass protest. Most animal activists have experienced at least some form of personal transformation and are now living an anti-speciesist, plant-based, or vegan lifestyle. Other forms of personal transformation include yoga, taking classes, and practicing a religion. Alternatives can include funding or operating an animal sanctuary, starting a YouTube channel, and creating a plant-based business. Inside game can mean running for political office, working within mainstream media outlets to get stories covered, or lobbying established political figures. Structure organizing is growing your network of activists and leaders to pressure those in power into bringing about change. Mass protest includes marches, lockdowns, and farm occupations.

Where to Start

If you have an idea for a unique organization, want to get involved with a protest group, or start a YouTube channel, my suggestion would be to get going ASAP. If you want to start a YouTube channel, for example, JUST START! There will never be a perfect moment, when you have all the right equipment, the best content, or the most viewers. You will figure out best practices along the way. Your audience, production value, and content will get better as long as you remain dedicated to and consistent with the project. You will get immersed in the broader community, acquire new ideas and perspectives, gather more resources, draw more of an audience, and gain more credibility as time goes on. Waiting for perfection, buy-in from the masses, or 100 percent support from everyone near you will have you waiting for an eternity. As long as your activism is nonviolent and is centered on the animals, your work will be a net positive for them.

"You're Making Us Look Bad! You're Doing More Harm Than Good!"

How many of us have heard this before? How many of us have used this against an organization or individual within the community? This type of rhetoric is extremely detrimental to the broader movement. Many of us already face incredible criticism for our life choices and activism, whether from our friends, our family, or society at large. The absolute last people we need to be receiving unwarranted criticism from are those from within the community.

These comments and sentiments are also further exacerbated by social media. There is no denying that since the advent of social media, dialogue in general has become more polarized. It's almost as if everything is a debate, and no one is willing to admit they're wrong. Some of the most viewed and viral content about animal rights happens to be footage of protests or acts of civil disobedience that has been either livestreamed or produced after the fact. It's worth noting that when someone leaves comments such as, "This is driving people away from the cause," or, "This is why people hate vegans," it is impossible to distinguish whether that person is vegan/plant-based or not. This should be cause for reflection. The corporations and business entities that exploit animals are very much united, as they have a vested interest in maintaining the status quo. How can we ever expect to dismantle speciesist systems when we ourselves are not united?

I firmly believe that those phenomena that are the most detrimental, toxic, and hindering to the animal rights movement occur within our own ranks, in the form of groups or individuals who 1) believe their way is the only way to achieve success and/or 2) condemn others for their form of activism or protest. I cannot stress how negative of an impact this rhetoric can have on the movement, especially on new or emerging activists.

What We Must Learn from History

When we think of Gandhi fighting for India's independence, the Pankhurst family championing women's suffrage, or Martin Luther King Jr. dreaming of a United States of America devoid of segregation, the commonality is clear: direct action and civil disobedience are a must. There has never been a successful movement for collective liberation that didn't have a mass protest element as part of the broader strategy.

No great change, awakening, or societal shift has ever taken place without radical activists taking to the streets, protesting, being loud, and getting arrested. It is important to note that many Black people during the civil rights movement did *not* agree with Dr. King and his methods of civil disobedience. There was much turmoil within the Black church related to the perceived effectiveness and validity of civil disobedience. Many claimed that marches, sit-ins, and other forms of civil disobedience made Black people as a whole "look bad" and believed these actions were "doing more harm than good." The fact that animal rights activists are now facing similar criticisms, inside and outside of the movement, is not surprising.

Both those within and those not within the ranks of animal rights also commonly argue that you "can't compare those previous movements with animal rights," that "it's different because those movements dealt with humans," or that "tactics historically used for human victims won't work for animals." While it is true that the experiences of the victims of various forms of systemic oppression throughout history have varied drastically, the underlying ideology that has enabled oppression is the same. So why would the path to liberation not be the same?

Remain Uncomfortable

In my few short years as an activist, I have sent emails, disrupted restaurants and grocery stores, been arrested, organized marches, and take part in undercover investigations. I have been praised and scorned by those within the ranks of animal rights for every one of these actions. Any action that we take is going to receive derision—from all sides! We must be prepared mentally to press on and use this misguided outrage as fuel to fire our activism.

If you yourself are not into activism, I encourage you to get involved. If you are already involved, I encourage you to try new things. If you've decided that activism is not for you, the least you can do is support those who are taking action. It is okay to be uncomfortable. In fact, we should strive to remain uncomfortable. The moment we get comfortable, we get complacent. Complacency will lead to the death of our movement. The death of our movement will result in the death of our planet. We cannot let this happen, so please, stay uncomfortable and get involved!

SECTION FOUR
Body and Spirit

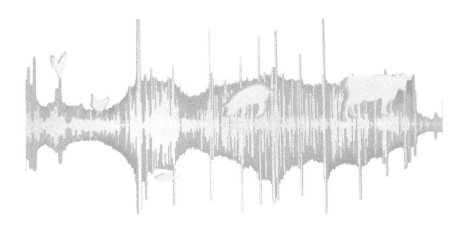

NANCY ARENAS

Vegan Activist, Event Coordinator,
Author, Publisher, Podcaster

Nancy Arenas is a vegan advocate and speaker, certified vegan nutrition coach, and the founder and organizer of Red & Green VegFest Albuquerque. She has authored the children's book *Wiatt the Vegan Pirate*, publishes the online magazine *New Mexico Vegan*, and as a vegan chef, shares recipes and dietary information through the group Cooking with Compassion. Her newly formed 501c3 nonprofit organization Sprouting Compassion will allow her to promote the vegan lifestyle full-time through events, programs, sponsorships, and donations. Nancy's goal is to create a more compassionate and cruelty-free world. Her personal mantra is: "Live with compassion, eat without violence."

A JOURNEY TO AN AWAKENING OF THE BODY, MIND, AND SOUL

I remember growing up in Brooklyn, New York, in the 1970s. I feel grateful that it was *my* generation fighting at the time for the environment ("Give a Hoot, Don't Pollute"), for women's rights ("Give Women Rights or We'll Fight"), for peace ("Make Love Not War"), for racial equality ("Don't Let Racism Divide Us"), and for animals ("Animal Liberation"). These slogans sound so familiar even now, and it's so distressing that we still need to speak up about the same issues today. We have not come so far from the seventies at all.

Why did I write the above? Because I was part of that generation fighting for the rights of all. As I reminisce, I cannot help but recognize that even though I was an activist then, I really had no clue what the word meant. It just seemed like the right thing to do for the planet, the people, and the animals. I understood that we needed to take care of our home, Earth. I understood that all humans should have the same rights, with no exceptions. I understood that women needed to be respected and not to be classified as "lesser than men"—I believed this not out of vengeance but because it was true. I did, genuinely and naturally, *feel* the certainty of all these principles, that rights existed for people, animals, and the planet. Though I believed in animal liberation, I did not truly comprehend what that really meant. After all, I loved animals then and I love them still. I enjoyed visiting the zoo, where I could see the beautiful animals, especially the lions, not realizing that it was a prison and that the animals did not belong there. As I said, I loved the animals, but I did not even consider what was on my plate. I guess I was taught, as most of us are, to love pets—cats, dogs, and other companion animals—but not to think about the other animals who are exploited. I lived thinking I was speaking up for animals, while I still ate them and supported such cruel entities as circuses, aquariums, and zoos.

Let us now move forward to what I call my "awakening." In 2013, I finally connected the dots. I finally was able to understand what an animal's existence means in animal agriculture: torture and suffering. Animal agriculture means *an animal's happiness is denied*. The suffering and death that animals endure at the hands of humans are grievous, nauseating, and exasperating. The fact that I had supported all this during all the years prior to my awakening made me feel not only deflated but also mad. It made me mad because society, family, and colleagues had all led me, like millions of others, down this path. They had robbed me of my compassion for all.

In 2013, after dealing with all this new information and my awakening, I felt I needed to act. I felt I had let the animals down long enough. It was time for me to truly rise up for the animals. I needed to step up for veganism. The question in my mind was how I could do this. How could I contribute?

I came across the Meatless Mondays campaign and created a petition through Care2 for Meatless Mondays in New Mexico. This was the beginning of my advocacy efforts. Unfortunately, the petition garnered only thirty-four supporters. I was disheartened, to say the least, but I was only made more passionate about spreading information on veganism. In my mind, I thought that if more everyday individuals knew about veganism and all it stood for, people would joyfully join the vegan movement. After all, veganism is about peace and compassion. Who could be against that? In October 2015, the first issue of the electronic magazine *New Mexico Vegan* was published. This was a way to distribute and share information about all aspects of veganism. As Mahatma Gandhi is believed to have once said, "In a gentle way, you can shake the world." That was what I set out to do. Now in its seventh year, *New Mexico Vegan* has had contributors from all over the world. These have included Dr. Michael Greger, Dr. Joel Kahn, Dr. Will Tuttle, Dr. Joanne Kong, and everyday vegans who are bringing about change in their own communities, such as Jacqueline Fonseca, Tammy Fiebelkorn, Ebony McCormick, Greg Lawson, among others.

I kept researching, reading, and learning more and more about veganism. I researched vegan activists, vegan physicians, and vegan groups. I was on a quest to absorb as much information as I could about all aspects of veganism. I could even give a personal testimony as to the benefits of a whole-food plant-based diet, having been cured of bursitis, joint swelling, migraines, and fibromyalgia a month after I had gone vegan. I truly believed in my heart (I still do) that as I broadened my compassion to include all animals, the universe would show its kindness back toward me. Given the health benefits I had received, my passion for educating the public expanded.

Being an event coordinator by profession, my next step to advocate veganism was a no-brainer. I founded and organized the Red & Green VegFest Albuquerque in 2016. The theme was: "Eat without violence." Not only that, but I also landed three spots on our local TV channel, KRQE. It was one of the first times—if not the first time—that veganism was mentioned on TV in New Mexico. *Yippee-ki-yay!* That first VegFest had wonderful presenters, such as JL Fields, Dr. Caroline Trapp, Keith McHenry, and others. Promoting veganism became so important to me that I have personally funded this event for five years now. It has not been easy, but it is that important to me. In 2020, I created a 501c3 nonprofit, Sprouting Compassion, that will take on the Red & Green VegFest Albuquerque event and several other programs to promote veganism in the community at large.

Fostering veganism is at the forefront of everything I do. So when I was asked by the manager of our local Natural Grocers if I would consider doing vegan cooking demos, without a thought, I said, "Yes!" Cooking with Compassion became a successful monthly event at Natural Grocers. Most of our Sunday events were standing room only, with the place packed with individuals seeking to transition to plant-based eating. These sessions were designed to teach people how to make "easy-peasy" vegan recipes in thirty or fewer minutes. The demos showed how to veganize all genres of food, and we even had several Cooking with Compassion segments on KRQE-TV.

Then came March 2020, when the world was turned upside down due to COVID-19. Everyone was locked down. No in-person events. Social distancing. Mask wearing. One would hope that the whole world would now come to understand the saying, "What happens to one happens to all." Living through this pandemic and all its restrictions, I had to rethink and change some of the things I had been doing to promote veganism. Cooking with Compassion was put on hold. The Red & Green VegFest Albuquerque went virtual.

Inspired by a Toastmasters project I'd done, I created a podcast. On April 5, 2020, the first episode of *Vegan Pulse* aired. The podcast became my new approach to promoting veganism. It introduces people from all over the world. The topics are wide-ranging and the guests are varied. They talk about how they came to veganism and discuss their products, companies, or projects; everyday vegans share their untold stories. All these stories are fascinating.

For me, veganism has been a journey to an awakening of the body, mind, and soul. An awakening of the body that led me to understand the benefits of a whole-food plant-based diet—which is optimal for health—to understand that eating animals is not healthy. An awakening of the mind, as I now recognize animals as individuals who can experience joy and fear, who have families and friends and want to live free from harm. An awakening of the soul, as my spirit is filled with a higher purpose, a higher mindfulness of love and the divine, a higher consciousness that implores *Ahimsa*—love, genuine care, and compassion for all living beings. Besides, who wants to ingest the tortured, suffering soul of an innocent being? When you eat an animal, you are ingesting all that grief, all that pain, and all that suffering into your body. I am so grateful for the awakening that veganism led me to. I am more at peace, more understanding, and more joyful now that I do not house a graveyard within me. Veganism is simply love—love for all.

Back in the seventies, I thought I was an activist. Now, I know—I am an activist for all sentient beings, human and nonhuman.

Let us resolve to exert ourselves heartily to propose the vegan ideal to all.

As we awaken to veganism, our compassionate outreach expands.

Voice "the pure vegan objective," for it is destined to be heard.

T. COLIN CAMPBELL, PHD

*Jacob Gould Schurman Professor Emeritus of
Nutritional Biochemistry, Cornell University*

T. Colin Campbell was trained at Cornell University (MS, PhD) and
MIT (Research Associate) in nutrition, biochemistry, and toxicology;
since 1975, he has been Jacob Gould Schurman Professor (now Emeritus)
at Cornell University. His principal scientific interests, derived from
his career in experimental research and policy making, concern the
fundamentals of nutrition. He is the recipient of several awards, both
in research and in citizenship. He has authored *The China Study* (2005,
co-authored with his son, Thomas M. Campbell, MD), *Whole* (2013,
with Howard Jacobson, PhD), and *The Future of Nutrition* (2020, with
Nelson Disla).

MAKING NUTRITION REAL

I am well into the ninth decade of my life and still learning more about
the vegan "movement." I first learned of vegetarianism when I was well
into my forties, while veganism came in my fifties. My initial points of
contact with these views were separate from the science in which I was
trained and working. In order to more fully understand that contact,
therefore, it's important that I explain my personal and scientific
background.

Long before I ever heard the word "vegetarian," I had been just a
kid on a dairy farm. I was raised milking cows, working the fields, and
harvesting crops, like generations of my family before. Except for when
I was in school, work was from sunrise to sunset, 365 days per year. In
those days, the school year in rural America was shorter than it is now,
lasting from Labor Day in September to about the first of May, because
we farm kids had chores to do at springtime.

Being the oldest son, I was given the responsibility of milking about twenty cows, using milking machines, although the first few years I only milked a couple cows by hand. In my limited spare time, I fished the stream in our meadow, hunted squirrels and rabbits, and for a few years trapped fur-bearing animals: muskrat and skunk. This was what farm boys did, and I loved it. I felt that our relationship with the outdoors was very close, as was our relationship with our animals. They weren't taken for granted and had names, and the cows had pedigrees. Even so, we sold cows at the local auction when they were too old for milking; we dehorned calves, castrated bull calves and pigs, and caponized male chicks; and we joined neighbors in the fall to butcher hogs.

My dad was an immigrant from Northern Ireland, and he had only had a couple of years of formal schooling before his family came through Ellis Island, but education was very important to him. When it came time for me to go to high school, he didn't want me to attend the local school because only about 10 percent of its graduates went on to college, mostly to be farmers or teachers. Instead, he arranged for me to attend a free public school in Washington DC, just over 50 miles away. I traveled those 100-plus miles every day for the next five years of school, traveling with my younger brother and sister during the later years. During the summers, it was back to milking cows, plowing the fields, "making" hay, threshing grain.

After high school, during which I had had the good fortune of coming under the tutelage of several teachers and counselors, I attended college at Penn State, majoring in pre-veterinary medicine. I received early admission to veterinary school at the University of Georgia, a program that I attended until a surprise Western Union telegram arrived near the end of my first year from a well-known professor, offering me a scholarship to attend graduate school at Cornell. I accepted the offer and earned my master's and doctoral degrees in animal nutrition and biochemistry. My doctoral research, broadly speaking, was designed to improve livestock production so that more people could have a greater access to protein, especially the "high-quality" protein of animals. I even taught Livestock Feeds and Feeding, the centerpiece of which was protein nutrition.

After two years of postdoctoral research at MIT, I accepted a faculty position in nutrition and biochemistry at Virginia Tech, where, in addition to my teaching biochemistry, I was asked to be the coordinator of a US State Department project in the Philippines to help resolve childhood malnutrition. Its main purpose was to increase consumption of protein, particularly "high-quality," animal-based protein.

Though I didn't give it much thought at the time, there was a pattern: in each of these phases of my personal and professional life, I was focused on animal protein—whether by drinking milk and eating eggs and meat during my youth, teaching livestock production and doing experimental research to improve protein production in grad school, or coordinating a project to improve protein consumption among malnourished children in the Philippines. That was, until I learned of an experimental animal (rat) study in India that suggested consuming animal protein could increase the risk of liver cancer (a second focus of mine)—findings that directly opposed what I personally and professionally believed at the time. What I thought I knew was, suddenly, under serious threat; questions had to be answered.

This was the initiative for my experimental research career. I obtained public funding from an NIH grant, which was repeatedly renewed every two to three years for the next twenty-seven years. Although I had initially wanted to determine whether animal protein increases cancer, I instead chose the research plan of using varying amounts of dietary protein to better understand the biochemistry of cancer development. I did not want to highlight the hypothesis that animal-based protein causes cancer because I knew that directly testing this cherished nutrient in that way could derail research funding. Thus, I tentatively accepted these early observations and began exploring the mechanisms by which cancer develops.

The results of the experimental animal studies were astounding. The many students and technicians in my research group and I were uncovering a number of biological mechanisms by which the protein effect works. As I looked for the *key* biochemical mechanism that could explain the animal protein effect, I came to learn that there is no *single* key. There is no single mechanism. Instead, there are many mechanisms that appear to work in harmony. For example, protein increases 1) carcinogen entry into the cell, 2) enzymatic activation of the carcinogen, and 3) a growth hormone that increases cancer cell development and the production of free radicals that encourage cancer growth. Simultaneously, it decreases 1) DNA repair that prevents mutation and 2) the immune system's production of natural killer cells, both of which are the body's natural defense against cancer. The ability of protein to increase cancer is clearly real, and there are multiple mechanisms we could point to in order to explain *how*. With such evidence mounting, we virtually could not refute the protein effect on cancer.

Follow-up studies proved to be even more far-reaching. We saw that other nutrients also use countless mechanisms to produce their effects and work together synchronously in order to create health and prevent disease. Animal protein (as casein) turns on cancer development; plant protein (such as soy, wheat) does not. We could turn cancer growth on or off simply by increasing or decreasing dietary animal protein. This remarkable distinction between animal and plant proteins is consistent with observational studies on humans: animal protein consumption, as reflected in the total diet, linearly increases with death rates for various cancers, heart diseases, and other degenerative diseases.

We also found evidence that undermined the widely held notion that cancer is a genetic disease. Our studies showed that although cancer is *initiated* by mutated genes, it is thereafter controlled by nutrition. Our ability to turn cancer growth off was exceptionally interesting because it suggested that disease might be *treated* by the same nutrition that prevents disease. A few years later, colleagues doing studies on diet and disease in humans showed that indeed, heart disease, Type 2 diabetes, chronic kidney disease, and many other ailments could be reversed or treated by reversing the nutritional exposures that promote them.

This multiplicity of nutrients—each nutrient by a multiplicity of mechanisms—acting both to prevent and to treat a broad spectrum of diseases suggested to me the concept of wholism (the "w" intended). This effect is apparent, as indicated by the maze of biochemical reactions that occur together within the trillions of cells in the body. The fact that these reactions interact with such harmony is truly amazing. It suggests that nutrition is not the summation of a certain number of nutrients acting independently. It also helps explain why single nutrients (and their drug cousins), in the absence of context, act differently, producing unwanted side effects.

As we delved deeper into the effects of protein and recognized the strikingly different effects of animal- and plant-derived proteins, it became abundantly clear that foods in the plant kingdom optimize health, while animal-based foods do the opposite. But also, their effects are complementary: as we consume more animal food, we consume less plant food.

When we compare the rates of disease (usually degenerative diseases) of different societies against group-specific indicators of animal and plant food consumption, we see these combined effects. For example, animal food consumption is estimated exclusively by animal protein and/or cholesterol, whereas plant food consumption is estimated exclusively by dietary fiber. Using these indicators, we see several very impressive linear correlations of degenerative disease rates with animal food consumption, all the way down to zero animal food intake. In other words, *any amount* of ingested animal food theoretically increases disease risk. This raises a serious question: why do we consume any animal-based food?

History contains numerous clues. Protein was chemically isolated for the first time from meat in 1839 and given its name from the Greek word *proteios*, meaning "of prime importance." Later, highly influential nutrition pioneers celebrated protein as "the stuff of life itself" and "the stuff of civilization." Although plant protein gradually appeared during the next half-century, it was considered to be of lower quality.

Ever since that auspicious baptism, animal-based protein has been so revered that scientists who dared to produce contrary evidence, no matter how reliable, risked their professional reputations. During the 1920s, this reverence was scientifically fixed when nutrition scientists began to measure the quality of individual proteins based on how efficiently they were retained in the body for *healthy* effects. Unfortunately, this perceived "biological value" ignores the *unhealthy* effects produced by the same proteins. Animal proteins, including the protein found in human flesh, are absorbed more completely and thus are considered "higher-quality"; they contribute to faster growth, but also to faster cancer growth as well as elevated blood cholesterol, which is associated with heart disease. On the other hand, plant-based proteins, which are not retained as well, are considered "low-quality."

Hidden between the lines of this history and beneath a great deal of pro-animal protein dogma is a very simple message: there is no nutritional need for animal-based protein; a whole-food, plant-based (WFPB) diet provides all the protein we need.

This is only a brief snapshot of my experience in experimental research. I am now abundantly convinced that the nutrition of a WFPB diet can create more health for more people than can all the pills and procedures now used. Not only did our research findings radically shift my views of nutrition, they also led my entire family (now twenty-four in number) to adopt this diet, thanks to my wife Karen, who created tasty foods that matched the research findings.

Perhaps unsurprisingly, my views and our research findings have often been equated with veganism and vegetarianism. However, though I accept and respect advocacy for the more humane treatment of animals, I have never deliberately aligned myself with these concepts. In fact, I have some reservations about them.

For one thing, I am troubled by the narrow approach of too many vegan advocates. While animal welfare is important, I am wary of viewing it—or, in fact, anything else—as the chief concern for all food choices. There are many factors to consider, and I worry that a focus so single-minded, no matter on what, tends to sidestep the other good reasons for dietary lifestyle change. Focusing exclusively on the ethical argument may detract not only from the less polarizing, fundamental science-based evidence that underlies food choices, but also from environmental problems that loom large, rising healthcare costs and the unequal distribution of healthcare, and the stagnation of authoritative institutions, public and private, that should be reformed to better serve the public. These problems are all interconnected; if the goal is to encourage broader change, as I believe it should be, then I think we should consider change in a broader sense.

For an example of this narrow-mindedness, consider the puzzling, self-destructive tendency of too many vegan advocates to ignore scientific evidence against animal protein, the most powerful evidence of all, solely because it has been produced in experimental animal (rodent) studies.

As much as I've tried to support the vegan community for at least 30 years—I've served on the medical advisory board of a prominent vegan group since its founding over 30 years ago and, during that time, invited several vegan leaders to lecture to my Cornell classes—I fear its argument against animal foods does not go far enough in meeting people where they are. As potentially noble as the ethical message may be, beginning with vegetarianism about 175 years ago, it has contributed to only a portion of total dietary change. I do not believe it alone will do enough to encourage change.

Even worse, vegan advocates shortchange their own cause by misreading the science of nutrition. For example, by assuming that human health problems are due to excessive intake of saturated fat and cholesterol, they deflect the powerful evidence against animal protein. This is unhelpful and confusing to the public, and gives animal industry enthusiasts something to dismiss as unsound science. One of the better known of the vegan activists, a member of the Vegetarian Hall of Fame, contacted me in 2013 to say that although he wanted to remain nameless, *The China Study* had done more to advance the cause of veganism than anything his vegan community had done. It was a generous gesture, and I appreciated his telling me to "keep it up," but it has been my impression both before and many times since that, bizarrely, much of the vegan community doesn't want to accept that very same evidence. Not all vegans, of course, but enough to make a significant difference.

Incidentally, I believe there are many good reasons to critique experimental animal research today, especially since we now have enough evidence to make the necessary decisions regarding human health and since the vast majority of such research is used for the evaluation of unnecessary candidate drugs. But this does not mean we can intentionally ignore the biological plausibility of core evidence questioning the eating of animals. Picking and choosing in that way do not make for a stronger argument.

The central theme of this book—cultivating personal empathy for all living creatures—reminds me of my own experiences working with seriously malnourished children in the Philippines and in Haiti. The inhumane conditions causing their plight begged for answers that I sought through science. The science led me in another direction— to question the evidence on animal protein, evidence that is now so convincing that it makes me wonder: *Why have we deceived ourselves so, for so long, about our need for protein that leads to the killing of 175 million cattle, 10 billion chickens, and 637 million pigs per year in the US alone?* We seek superior health but get early death combined with huge expenses. Though many things have changed between my working with those children and arriving at this fact, what concerns me most is what has not changed: there remain a serious lack of empathy for all sentient beings and, it seems, a deficit of common sense.

I acknowledge Nelson Disla for his editorial oversight.

CHATILLA VAN GRINSVEN

Professional Athlete and Animal Rights Advocate

Chatilla van Grinsven is a Dutch world-class professional basketball player. She has accumulated numerous honors throughout her career, including as an A-10 Conference champion, French Cup champion, Big-5 Player of the Year, and winner of the Roosevelt Hunter Community Service Award. In the US, she was nominated for the NCAA Woman of the Year Award. Van Grinsven has a bachelor's degree in international business from Saint Joseph's University and a master's degree in global diplomacy from the University of London. Today, Chatilla is an active advocate for human and animal rights and is determined to use her platform as a voice for the voiceless. She is an ambassador for the Dutch political party *Partij voor de Dieren* (Party for the Animals).

MY JOURNEY TO CREATING A MORE COMPASSIONATE WORLD

My journey of awareness started in 2016, when I got a puppy. Her name is Luna, and she is now five years old. She is a sweet golden retriever and travels with me everywhere I go in the world for my basketball career. I've traveled and lived with her in the most diverse, dynamic, and beautiful places around the globe, such as France, Turkey, the US, the Netherlands, Italy, and many other places. Luna has become my best friend; wherever I go, she is there. We have become such a team—so connected—that we are often compared to characters in the amazing movie *Hachi: A Dog's Tale*. She walks without a leash and understands exactly what I mean with just a few words. She stops, she sits, she walks by my side all on command or at a signal of my hand. Our communication is 90 percent nonverbal, and that is the true language of life, for all living beings can be understood if you just connect with them through the soul. Connecting with Luna was what started my journey to compassion and understanding and opened up my eyes to the world and all its beautiful living creatures, whether they walk, swim, or fly upon this earth. I started to understand that we are *all* the same. We call ourselves "humans" and other living beings "animals," but at the end of the day, all living beings have feelings and an understanding of nature. We are all creatures; we are all "animals." Just because we don't speak the vocal languages of other species does not mean we cannot connect with them, feel compassion for them, or understand them.

Almost all of us grow up eating meat, wearing leather, and consuming other types of animal products; I did, too. We never consider the impact on the animals involved. It was only during this past decade that more attention started to be focused on the shocking animal agriculture industry, wherein animals are abused and used to meet the market's demand for animal products. It has become such a large, lucrative industry that animals are exploited and seen as "products" instead of living beings with families and feelings of their own.

Ever since I was a little girl, I have had a deeply rooted connection to nature, animals, and life as a whole. I remember, at a young age, speculating philosophically about the meaning of life and what we as individuals have come here to do. I remember, on car rides to basketball practice, looking outside the window and seeing all the wonderful trees and plants, and animals roaming around, thinking how beautiful life is. I was still very young at that time, probably around fourteen years old, going through life happy, mesmerized by the beauty of all that life has to offer and all that life is. You could say that as children, we have a certain degree of tunnel vision, whereby much of the real world is blocked out; this remains very true even as we become grown-ups. What we see around us, including all the information we receive from mainstream media, becomes our reality. Seeing through tunnel vision becomes a way of living, and large parts of the truth are hidden away to make way for a more comfortable reality. This is especially the case with the animal agriculture industry, which, with comfortable indifference, hides the barbaric conditions in which the animals live and then are slaughtered at the end of their shortened lives. This is done so consumers do not associate a piece of meat with the cruelty and pain the animal underwent. Today, the truth is exposed in many eye-opening documentaries, such as *Cowspiracy* by Kip Andersen. As I watched this film, the facts behind the consumption of meat and other animal products were suddenly revealed to me. Although these facts are now much more of a topic of discussion in the general media, there is still an urgent need to expose them further. The way we treat animals has an immense impact not only on these beings of unique beauty and intellect, but also on the wellbeing of our own planet. Our existence, and especially that of future generations, are directly affected.

The choice we make today is one that will impact all of us in other ways as well, such as in many aspects of our health. This is a journey of awareness. During the last few years, I have become aware of the pain we cause animals throughout their entire lives by choosing to consume animal flesh and other animal products. I now *consciously* choose what I eat, knowing the impacts that my meals have on other sentient beings. When I started to consume delicious plant-based options that are not only incredibly tasty but also full of high-value nutrition, I started to notice my performance level as a professional athlete go up as well. Before that, I had had no idea that it would affect my health in such an incredible way, in such a short time. I also noticed I needed a lot less sleep and overall felt extremely fit at a consistent level. Overwhelming scientific evidence shows that eating meat and other animal products can cause obesity, high cholesterol, and high blood pressure, in turn increasing the risk of heart and cardiovascular disease. Yet this is not the only downside of meat consumption. The inhumane way in which animals are treated in the factory farming industry causes them great distress.

I often pass through a farm neighborhood near my house when I go for long walks with Luna. We always pass by various farms with several acres of land. The owner of one of the largest farms has a stable that is packed with roughly four hundred cows in extreme confinement, with only a few feet of space between them to move around. One day, I decided to talk to the farmer and ask why the cows were all crammed together inside—why he was not using his many acres of land to let the cows graze and roam freely. He stated, very rationally, "It is more cost-efficient; the cows can be milked faster if they always stand in close proximity to the milk machine." I was shocked by his answer, but it is the sad truth. This industry is all about business and not about the animals. But it is also a fact that we, with our own food choices, can turn this around. In the animal agriculture industry, animals are enslaved and used as products for us to wear, eat, and drink. The industry is characterized by a sense of entitlement and absolutely no remorse, even as it artificially inseminates a cow and takes her newborn baby away, ignoring her heartbreaking cries that last for days—all so consumers can put milk on their cereal. If the calf is a baby boy, the usual routine is for him to be sent to the slaughterhouse or raised for veal. If the calf is a baby girl, she will face the same fate as her mother—being impregnated several times in her life and losing her babies to the industry. Once her body is spent from producing milk, when she is only about five or six years old, she, too, will be sent to the slaughterhouse. However, in today's world, we have the luxury of replacing beef burgers with plant-based burgers and cow's milk with plant-based milk, both of which are after all a lot healthier, too.

When we are able to understand that all animals feel emotions, we will be able to end speciesism. We are all creatures, as different on the outside as we are similar on the inside. We all bleed the same; we all experience similar sensations when we are happy, or scared and hurt. All species deserve to live free from suffering, harassment, and oppression. I believe Joaquin Phoenix, in his Academy Awards speech on February 9, 2020, summed it up in the best possible way:

> I think at times we feel, or we're made to feel, that we champion different causes. But for me, I see commonality. I think whether we're talking about gender inequality or racism or queer rights or indigenous rights or animal rights, we're talking about the fight against injustice. We're talking about the fight against the belief that one nation, one people, one race, one gender, or one species has the right to dominate, control, and use and exploit another with impunity.

I have to say that one of my life's absolutely happiest and most fulfilling moments happened in 2020, when I was able to save a beautiful piglet's life. I remember that day well: I had received an email response from Melief Sanctuary in the Netherlands, telling me that there was room at the sanctuary for one pig. I drove up right away to meet one of the sanctuary's founders, and we visited every pig farm in the neighborhood to talk to the farmers, with the intention to save one of the pigs. Most of the farmers either were not at home or rejected our request, but we did not give up. We kept talking to farmers in the neighborhood to share our point of view and see if someone would let us have one pig. Finally, the sixth farmer we spoke to let his guard down and was willing to give us a pig after our entreaties. I remember it was at the end of the afternoon when we brought the piglet (now named Chati) to the sanctuary. On the way back, we passed by a slaughterhouse where, every day, fifteen thousand pigs are killed at the age of only six months. Chati was only three months old at the time; in a few months' time, she would have ultimately ended up there with her brothers and sisters. I remember feeling powerless from not being able to save those thousands of other lives, but Chati the piglet will forever be the symbol of a freedom fighter in her community, representing all those other beautiful individuals who did not make it. She now roams around and lives a life full of freedom and joy with her new pig friends at Melief Sanctuary—the "land of the free."

We have the power to use our voices for the voiceless and to stop the inhumane slaughtering of animals for human consumption. We human beings are so incredibly smart, inventive, creative, and ingenious. When we choose compassion and love for all species to guide our lives, we will be able to invent and implement innovative systems that benefit our own health, sustain the planet, and value all sentient beings.

If there is one valuable lesson you could take away from this essay, it is that all living species on our planet are connected to each other, for we are all distinctively equal and are in turn equally connected to nature. We all live in an ecosystem that we cannot escape from, and therefore, we have to treat it with care, respect, and a certain level of compassionate consciousness. Consequently, though we often defer responsibility to our governments, NGOs, or activists, we all have a personal responsibility to take action right now, every day of our lives—to vote with our wallets as we choose which products to buy. I strongly believe in the power of awareness to allow us to live a healthier and more conscious lifestyle—for ourselves, the planet, and of course, the animals. My journey of awareness has allowed me to joyfully choose a plant-based life. I strongly believe that the art of living lies deeply rooted in the conscious mind; to tap into it, we need only have the courage to explore and choose to change for the better.

Dr. Elisa Beth Haransky-Beck

Vegan Optometrist and Environmentalist,
OD, MA, PDC, SMT

Dr. Elisa Beth Haransky-Beck has been a holistic vision practitioner for over thirty-three years, specializing in natural vision improvement. She facilitates positive change through her work as a vegan optometrist, somatic movement therapist, veganic permaculturist, spiritual nutrition counselor, yogini at EmbodyVision, and organizer of Vegan Spirituality-Southwest PA. Author of *Enlivening Consciousness*, Dr. Haransky-Beck founded the Schwartz Living Market in Pittsburgh, Pennsylvania, an early demonstration project of living foods and living buildings. Her home in Monroeville, Pennsylvania, features a veganic permaculture landscape.

The Terrain

Moving through these unprecedented times by moving within The stories of competition are melting away into stories of being ness in cooperation and collaboration And these stories begin by coming back to the clarity of ourselves Moving Within Vibration

New Beginnings Beginning with what we put into our mouths each day in the form of food and water And with how we Breathe Cellular breath

Re-membering
Moving toward or completely into purity and then more easily allowing the flow of purity and grace and oneness to flow through us untethered—free from head to tail to fingers and toes through a free Spine with full breath

Beginning

Beginning again With the Sprouts that contain all of the enzymes and nutrients to begin again

Fresh Renewed Rejuvenated Beginning from where we are without judgment Where do we begin? Within!

Meditation several times a day Finding our true authentic natures and knowing why we are here in these incredible moments in this form

Based in Real Food Veganism Cooperation *Collaborating* in *Family* in *Community with Spirit*

With our Breath Breathing Ourselves fully
The dura of the brain The crura of the thoracic and pelvic diaphragms
The unified diaphragms of our selves and breathing as one being and then with all of every thing As One

Participating in Tikkun Olam: Repairing the World—by beginning within.
The Becoming: A back and forth Spiralic in Nature Process Ebb and Flow On the Go
We are all Becoming Moving into our ideal selves Gradually or immediately In the way we are meant to unfold In the way we are meant to BE.

Veganism Permaculture Agriculture Carnism Carnivore
Herbivore Monoculture Visionary Luminary Embodiment Discretionary

Respect Self-Respect Enlivening Consciousness Innovation Creation
Embodied with Breath and Spirit Spirited

Transformation Transmutation Alchemy Alchemizing Alchemizing the dissonance

The separation The differences
Moving Into the realization we are it is all ONE One-ness

The bees the birds the trees
The microbes we are made of
The bats the insects the anteaters
The microbiome is our inner ecosystem The Terrain
The worms the snakes the lizards Inside of us we co-mingle with all
that is was and ever will be We are one We are that which is Inside
and outside of us The Terrain
We are nature Our inner nature and that which we perceive lies
outside of us
We are not separate as we have educated ourselves into We are our
embodied visionary selves
When we eat animals we are eating the cells of ourselves
Where did this understanding or lack of understanding come from?
The disconnect is a deeply cultural construct
Deconstruction
Look around Blame others And then realize how we externalize How
we seem to think feel and act as if the issues are "out there"
Where?
Inside Inside We must GO Go INSIDE Inside into the inner
ecosystems of the souls of our microbiomes Deep Deep Deep
inside Take a ride with ourselves Into the realm of our unconscious
subconscious knowingness

When we eat animals we're eating ourselves
The karma The thoughts The DNA and RNA and Soul of other beings

How did we land here? Why did Spirit allow us to take this course?
And with every season turn turn turn There is a season and a reason.
Or is there?
I know this to be true for me All of it—All of the disconnect from
myself and my true nature The way I tortured and abused my body
Through the years the trainings the ballet The coursework the "tests"
Thinking Thinking Thinking over-riding the BEING
Where are we now? In the middle of the transformative moments

Enlightenment The Apocalypse of Choices Choosing Choosing to live
in harmony with nature
To truly SEE To let go of destructive habit patterns from deep within
our collectively conscious soul First to integrate and assimilate and
know that our histories our herstories and our they and theirstories
have Flowed through us But now The time has come to tell and feel
And BE the new Way

What's old is new again The rising The arising Of our true natures as
one with ourselves and that which is within is without consuming meat
and chickens and fishes and milks from animals
The divine feminine and the divine masculine rising within all of
us. Where the borders are fluid and permeable and pure Where the
gunk has been loosened so much that it flows and dissipates The pure
reabsorption revolution And we integrate our understanding that we
knew not what we were doing when we were eating all that dead flesh
and the milk of animals meant for their own young and the eggs meant
to turn into animals

The pinnacle of agribusiness including In the world of "kosher" has
passed It's over It's done But that's not all We're calling ourselves
out on all levels—because none of us-not yet-can truly call ourselves
"vegan" Why? Animal products are contained everywhere—In this
Anthropocene era—we see the carnage all around The plastics of the
dinosaurs The inner ecosystem pollution of microplastics and synthetic
nanoparticles—and the wondering of why we feel so sick

Why we have to work so hard to PURIFY and boost our immunity. Or
do we? What is purity integrity wholesomeness? The myth that we can
rise above all that surrounds us
The urgency creating dissonance When all there is really is the
RIGHT NOW
Where are we? Do we know our place? Do we have a place in this
space called EARTH?

Are we ready to Ascend into our true natures with the understanding that WE are all that we have been waiting for We are right where we need to be In the Now

Hineni: Here I am. Here we are. What will we choose?

Choice. The choice is ours to create the new beautiful joyful harmonious melodious embodied selves that we know deep in our hearts and souls we have always been
The day is here where we do not fear ourselves or the other Where we see and act and think and feel in harmony with all that is was and ever will be

And letting go into the letting in of the flow of nature the humaneness the humanness huwomanness the divine feminine and divine masculine of the humanity of our strength Integrity and open true natures

Diving diving Deep Ready Set Go!

We know the bee The bee
BZZZZ
With the bee We see The Buzz We know it We hear it
We are THAT We are ONE And we see ourselves We are done externalizing

There is pain There is dissonance And then You know Integrate And let it go into the nothing

Eat those plants—sentient or not The next level of Beingness in its depth is here
We have arrived to not simply survive But THRIVE!
Ahhh—the beauty the breadth Breathe deeply with depth The depth of the deep embodied Knowingness within

We do not erase the experiences of the past Yet—the collective consciousness through its own understanding and the help of angels and the helper beings in the universe are here for us and with us and through us We are rising into the EN LIGHT EN MENT in the present tense And so it is

Here and Now The proclamation of transmutation with the critical masses The inner terrain informing and forming what's next

The miracle of 2020 and here we are Here we go And so it is And so it is And so it IS The IS The ISNESS of the Organic Veganic Living Foods Permaculture Integration Reinvention Revolution inside and out and all around Ahhhhhhh: We're Alive as ONE!

With Deep Gratitude to Dr. Joanne Kong for her deep insights in creating this anthology and for seeing in me through the bee and the sunflower

GISELLE MEHTA

Vegan Writer and Speaker

Giselle Mehta is a vegan advocate whose versatility stems from her drawing upon her diverse creative abilities as a noted writer, speaker, and entrepreneur. In demand for her soulful insights, she speaks on a variety of subjects at numerous public events. She was a co-owner of Carrots, India's first all-vegan restaurant. She advances the vegan cause through social events, the performing arts, and animal rescue activities, and with food, fashion, and personal care products. Giselle blogs on *Vegan-Elle* and is author of the novel *Blossom Showers*. For a decade, she served the Indian Revenue Service in a senior capacity.

THE ROAD TO A HIGHER SELF

Being vegan demonstrates a victory of the self over social conditioning. Forks in the personal pathway may converge to a destination of profound personal awakening. Proclivities of the pre-vegan self can progress to new potential and deeper engagements. Compassionate connection with all beings may raise one to yet higher consciousness. Here is a personal epic. . . .

The Starting Point

Our family contemplated an issue with potentially grim consequences. The "why" of the situation bewildered us, for we lived ethically according to most tenets. We extended our welfare activities to nonhumans as well, being mindful of shelter and street animals. Always one to ponder deeply on things to find analytic solutions, I experienced an insightful eureka moment. It struck me that merely doing good isn't enough. One must also avoid inflicting hurt and harm beyond the human circle, limits normally considered sufficient for moral restraint. The starting point would be to stop the pain and bloodshed we cause our fellow living beings through our meal choices, whereby we use our wallets to merely delegate the knifework to professional entities.

As I was responsible for the meals on the table, my strategy of mastering the dietary shift with tasty plant-based alternatives also turned other family members vegan. From a starting point of eliminating cruel and expropriatory foods, I expanded the exclusions to leather, silk, and general consumer items that leave a trail of animal suffering behind them. The issue that had elicited my epiphany transformed into a positive outcome—a vegan lifestyle that shuns hidden violence. Treating all beings as worthy of life, I felt more authentic in my claim to being an animal lover.

The Stepping Stones

I've enjoyed a versatile life, doing different things. People acquainted with various aspects of my persona may be surprised to find that ardent vegan activism now shapes my core. However, my past and current immersions have been preparatory or complementary to this crucial evolution of my being.

In my teens, I was an enthusiastic quizzer, accumulating interesting and disconnected facts, winning trophies at public contests. My appetite for information led me to discover the catalogue of cruelties visited upon our nonhuman friends. Facts would now coherently connect to form larger pictures that link animal suffering, ecological crises, and human disease.

I pursued a master's degree at a famous Indian university known for its radical outlook. The thinking there continues to be anthropocentric, focused on a limited section of human interests. Where my university experience shaped me is in my willingness to take on an unjust status quo. The shift to compassionate consumption represents resistance to corporate systems centered on suffering and environmental devastation, which often misrepresent themselves as being benign and healthful.

My working life started in the Indian bureaucracy. Though it was a job that demanded a stiff persona, performing important public functions at a relatively young age (from my mid-twenties to my thirties) left me feeling responsible for the vulnerable everywhere. I find it unbearable to be a passive bystander to inequity and injustice. There is currently no injustice remotely equal to the plight of voiceless animals, with both stupefying numbers and horrendous suffering. I believe that each awakened person, whether or not they are in a position of power, can be a leader within their respective circle to lead the way for transformational change.

After a decade in bureaucracy, I gravitated toward entrepreneurship. Amid the multiple engagements, my being co-owner of Carrots, a pioneering vegan restaurant in India, demonstrated a passion for bringing about positive change. Carrots was conceived as a system of support and inspiration and a venue for vegans and nonvegans alike to savor the flavors of plant-based eating, the first of its kind in the Indian public space.

Fertile Fields

Simultaneously, I am a published author who writes fiction. An author must enter the skin of a character to write a plausible story. A parallel to this is getting into the skin of animals in real life—gauging their terror and the torment they undergo in dairies, butcheries, laboratories, zoos, and sporting arenas. Each being is the bearer of a unique story and is deserving of recognition as an individual, not a commodity. In addition, I've found songwriting to be a creative activity with potential for wider reach. I've found using my voice to highlight animal suffering enhances the worth of words and the convergence of the creative arts, thus propagating a paradigm shift.

From "walking the talk," one may progress to "talking the walk." I use the public podium to reach diverse audiences that otherwise have never heard the merest whisper about veganism. I am a speaker, with a focus on the motivational side, at vegan events. It's even more interesting when I get to weave the narrative of veganism into general public events and articulate veganism's imperatives from an unusual point of convergence. For example, I vividly recall the audience being shocked when my talk on women and the environment unexpectedly put the ecological villainies of animal agriculture in the spotlight. At a Youth Power event, I urged a college audience to become changemakers for social justice; and speaking at an alumni event, I integrated veganism into the narration of my personal journey. At the release event for a book on Gandhi, I spoke of The Vegan Society, whose pioneering founders were inspired by Gandhian ideals of truth and nonviolence.

I also leverage my social persona for advocacy of a different kind. Parties and gatherings are an opportunity for me to show that a vegan diet can be varied, delicious, and nutritious. I organize potlucks where vegans and aspiring vegans can interact. I am a mentor in online groups, both local and global, that promote veganism.

Climbing the Mountain

Veganism propelled me into a lifestyle of self-reliance, with a preference for a do-it-yourself approach to vegan alternatives to animal products. This self-reliance has extended to other areas. Since my awakening drew on faiths emphasizing nonviolence, I gravitated toward Reiki as a healing alternative to cruel and suspicious pharmaceutical solutions. As an energetic form of healing, it led me to the next level of awakening: the realization that the physical universe is not as inanimate as we may presume. This converges with ongoing validation from quantum physics that our thoughts and words create our realities and contribute to the subtle energy grid of the universe. Healing is not only about alleviating individual ills. One may employ healing as complementary to other forms of activism to effect changes at the level of society's collective consciousness.

Sanskrit *mantras* form part of my regular spiritual practice. They are vibratory chants drawing on concepts that define deities of the Hindu pantheon. I continually discover how their subtle energies work to manifest desirable outcomes. For example, invoking the powerhouse of Shiva is aiming for a consistent regeneration of the needful and the positive. A chant to Goddess Saraswathi appeals for wisdom to make the world a kinder place. A simple chant aimed at the happiness of all (human and nonhuman) is: *"Loka Samastha Sukhino Bhavanthu."*

It's equally possible to set vibratory processes in motion with affirmations in one's familiar language that resonate. It's important that such affirmations read like something that is ongoing or already accomplished. The tone must be optimistic; negative realities must be rephrased into positive aspirations. An affirmation I have composed reads like this:

> I seek and receive good energies of the universe for blessings and healing for all beings—that they are safe and secure (whether amid nature or among humans); that they are supported in their needs, relieved of ills and injuries, saved from difficult situations and systems; and that innovation consistently directs systems toward compassion and conservation. Good energies support individual vegans to stay the course and power the growth of veganism everywhere. Production and consumption systems align to be universally beneficial. The earth and all her creatures benefit from human restraint and prudence. Compassion and kindness are growing forces for good that transform individuals and societies.

My immersions have attuned me to the idea that the body is a miniature universe, internally delineated by energy clusters called *chakras*. The Solar Plexus Chakra represents the sun and equates to the digestive system, which generates bodily energy for each individual from food intake. The sun is the source of photosynthesis in plants, which form the base of the food chain. In my thinking, compared to consuming animal products higher up in the food chain, eating a plant-based vegan diet allows one to directly access life-giving energy that nourishes mind, body, and spirit.

Human beings embody intelligent energy, with added capacities for feeling and doing.

Self-correction and constructive action are completely within our scope. This links up with two important practices in the Indian way: yoga and meditation. An important principle of yoga is *ahimsa* or nonviolence, because controlling our consumption leads to the energy shift that is self-mastery. To me, meditation is more than an energy practice; it is expanded consciousness that is connected with a living universe. The heartbeat of the universe is in all living beings, and we fulfill the spirit of meditation when we respect their right to live. I am connected with Brahmarishi Mohanji, a guru who propagates *ahimsa* and veganism. His various meditations, such as "Blossoms of Love" and "Power of Purity," honor the common energy principle that unites all beings.

The first few years of being vegan filled me with enormous tumult—from helpless rage against what happens to animals and anger toward those who perpetuate evil systems or willfully participate by way of consumption. I can feel meditative and healing practices leading me to a more evolved state. Being calmer in my being enables me to better radiate the inner peace that embodies the true vegan spirit. It may be a highly subjective experience, but one may draw connections between this kind of energy work and discernible progress in the growth of veganism and compassion. Being vegan is no longer a lonely journey, as seen by the rising numbers of vegans and celebrities adding heft to the cause. Even the catastrophe of a global pandemic, believed to have originated from meat markets, has furnished its own impetus toward plant-based eating. The whole world may not immediately abandon millennia-old patterns, but there is hope, as more individuals and food systems evolve in response to each other. More individuals who are open to their energetic potential to manifest good can accelerate the movement toward a more compassionate world.

Sighting the Peak

There have been times when I regretted not pursuing other career trajectories, but I feel gratitude for my current existence. I had to travel along a certain route of life to turn vegan, which is a high point in itself. Disconnecting from violent consumption choices creates peace and positivity at the level of subtle consciousness. A compassionate awakening of this nature is a road to the higher self.

VICTORIA MORAN

*Author, Podcaster, and Director, Main Street
Vegan Academy*

Listed among *VegNews* magazine's "Top 10 Living Vegetarian Authors" and voted PETA's "Sexiest Vegan Over 50" in 2016, Victoria Moran has written thirteen books, including *The Love-Powered Diet, Main Street Vegan*, and the international bestseller *Creating a Charmed Life*. Featured twice on *Oprah*, she hosts the award-winning *Main Street Vegan Podcast*, produced the 2019 documentary *A Prayer for Compassion*, and is director of Main Street Vegan Academy, training vegan lifestyle coaches and educators. A vegan of thirty-seven years, Victoria lives in New York City with her husband, Rev. William Melton—co-founder of The Compassion Consortium, a vegan ministry—and their rescue dog Forbes and rescue pigeon Thunder.

VEGANISM, YOGA, AND ME

From the time I heard the word "vegetarian" at age five, I knew there was something there for me, but I wouldn't find out what it was in 1950s Kansas City, with its eponymous steak and barbecue and massive stockyards. Still, "vegetarian" stayed in my head. Other exotic terms accumulated over time—"mysticism," "meditation," "yoga," "intuition," "reincarnation"—until I had a collection of out-of-reach concepts, each joined with the others in connoting the aspirational and the magical.

After high school, I moved to London, hung out with Quakers and Spiritualists, and spent every spare minute in a shop near Trafalgar Square—Watkins, "specializing in new, used, and antiquarian books in the mind, body, and soul field." I found a yoga teacher and stopped eating land animals. A year later, I was vegetarian in earnest and continued with yoga. Veganism took longer, but when I got there, I was still doing yoga—off and on as for the physical practice, but always "on" in the way I looked at life. And ever since, whatever I've done, wherever I've lived, and regardless of the priorities of the moment—school, marriage, parenthood, career—my companions have been yoga and veganism.

It may be hard to conceive of a time when it was considered avant-garde, rebellious, even sacrilegious to eat foods now available at standard supermarkets or to take up a fitness practice now offered at any Y. My mother noted how things had changed when, in her eighties, she said to me: "We used to think you were crazy, doing that yoga and eating those beans. But now, people's doctors tell them to do that." Indeed, they do, and yet I'm sufficiently rebellious and drawn to the avant-garde that even if the doctors said to do something different, I would not change.

I came into this life with a yogic worldview. I felt certain that I'd lived before and that God takes up residence within every living being. It always seemed to me that life on Earth is not the ultimate reality but nevertheless important, and I needed to do my best at it. As I learned that there are different religious faiths, it only made sense that each is there to lead its followers back to a collective home that belongs to us all. These odd notions were nurtured by my slightly eccentric, grandmother-aged nanny Adelene DeSoto (I called her Dede), who taught me most of the words on my exploration list. The others I gleaned largely from a fictional role model, Mame Dennis—*Auntie Mame*—in the classic motion picture starring Rosalind Russell.

In the movie, Mame celebrates diversity and tantalizing ideas in the 1920s; by the final scene, she is an elegant woman of a certain age who is about to take her great-nephew to India to visit her favorite yogi. "Have him back by Labor Day," the parents insist. "Labor Day," she muses, guiding her charge up a circular staircase, "that's sometime in November, isn't it?" Between Dede and Auntie Mame, there was no way I could take up grilling burgers and playing golf, even though my biological parents enjoyed both.

So there I was, eating funny and spending a lot of time upside down. It made for a glorious youth and middle age, but it's really only in my third act that I'm coming to see the immense value of a yogic vegan life. This way of being in the world demands a degree of rigor. I'm lazy and self-indulgent by nature, and without veganism and yoga, I might have long ago perished in a diner, missing both dessert and a playoff on *Jeopardy!*

As it is, the disciplines imposed by veganism and yoga have, to date, saved me. I've long understood the basic edicts of veganism to be: 1) consider the welfare of others, irrespective of species, in all your choices, and 2) prioritize the wellbeing of your arteries over the cravings of your palate. (I realize that nowadays, we often regard ethical vegans and plant-based health seekers as separate groups, separate movements even. When I started on this path, in the 1970s, however, most vegans made their choice for the animals but rapidly signed on to some iteration of "healthy eating." We had to prove that respect for animals wouldn't lead to sickness for humans. Back then, "eat your veggies" was as much a moral imperative as a nutrition tip.)

Next up are the disciplines of yoga, a sort of Ten Commandments in two parts, starting with the *yamas* or moral precepts:

- non-harming (even non-yogic vegans know this word in Sanskrit, *ahimsa*);
- truthfulness;
- non-coveting;
- restraint of the senses; and
- non-possessiveness.

These are followed by the *niyamas* or observances:

- cleanliness;
- contentment;
- discipline;
- study of oneself and spiritual teachings; and
- surrender to a higher power.

When I see these spelled out, I think I'm the sorriest would-be yogi who ever assumed a Downward-Facing Dog. Still, every day I show up, and some days I do better. Being vegan helps me at least to get a passing grade in *ahimsa*.

And I remain intrigued and inspired by the graceful interplay of veganism and yoga. It's in the teachings of the sages:

> Those noble souls who practice meditation and other yogic ways, who are ever careful about all beings, who protect all animals, are the ones who are actually serious about spiritual practice.—*Atharva Veda*, verse 19.48.5

> Just serve every living being in God's creation with humility, respect and love.—Neem Karoli Baba, spiritual teacher of Ram Dass

> A perfect action is one that does no harm to anyone and does some good for someone.—Swami Satchidananda, founder of Integral Yoga

And it's in yoga's practical philosophy, including its guidance on how to live, even how to eat. Yoga teaches that there are three modes or *gunas* governing life on Earth: *rajas* (passion), *tamas* (inertia), and *sattva* (goodness). They're all necessary. *Rajas* builds families and cities and civilizations. *Tamas* lets us sleep at night and allows for the death and decay that nourish the soil and the forests. But if you're looking to build character or sanctify your soul, you want to focus on *sattvic* practices—meditation, good deeds, time spent being in nature or otherwise surrounded by beauty, and engagement in spiritual discourse or immersion in spiritual study.

In addition, some foods are *sattvic* and contribute to both physical health and spiritual growth: fruits, vegetables, grains, legumes, nuts, and seeds. The ancient texts include "milk from healthy cows," but I contend that a cow in a dairy herd is unlikely to be healthy and is assuredly unhappy. Since dairying sentences cows and their calves to an untimely death, *ahimsa* is impossible to achieve when there's yogurt in the fridge and pizza in the freezer, unless these are vegan.

So I live each day habituated to teachings from a foreign land and a way of eating and of relating to nonhuman beings that is foreign to my Midwestern roots. Even so, these teachings fit me as if made to order.

In this era of cancel culture and online chastisement, I run the risk of a cultural appropriation charge. My rebuttal would be that I appropriated these beliefs and practices so long ago, I'm not sure where they stop and where I start. In my life, veganism and yoga have contributed as much to who I am as has my genetic code. They so infuse my life with meaning, purpose, and delight that I feel a bit like a carnival barker, armed with a pressure cooker and a sticky mat, calling out to passersby: "Step right up! Get your vegan yoga here. Believe me, ladies and gents, boys and girls: you don't want to miss out on this one."

NANCY POZNAK

Health Educator, MS, CHES, and Founder,
BotaniCuisine, LLC

Nancy Poznak is a health educator and the founder of BotaniCuisine: Plant-Sourced Dining Outreach. She has a master's degree in health science with a focus on community health education. Her background includes professional certification as a personal trainer, group fitness instructor, and health coach. Prior to studying health science, Nancy worked as a graphic designer and was an art director for *Muscle & Fitness* magazine. She founded BotaniCuisine to help increase plant-based/vegan food options in restaurants. She organized Baltimore's first Vegan Burger Smackdown in 2019 and founded Plant-Powered Meat Month, a promotion featuring restaurants and professional chefs. She also hosts vegan dining and social-interactive events and the monthly virtual meetup series *Plant-Powered: An Extraordinary Life*. Nancy has also created and given presentations titled "Many Reasons Vegan" and "Nutrition and Brain Function."

AWAKENING TO COMPASSION ACROSS THE DECADES

Growing up in a middle-class home and a typical suburban American family (with Mom, Dad, a brother, and a dog) long before cell phones and the Internet, I wasn't exposed to a wide range of perspectives and customs. Dinnertime was family time; shared meals helped strengthen emotional bonds and, as a family ritual, provided structure. Like almost everyone I've known, I never thought much about or questioned what we ate, how the food got to our plates, or how different foods affected our health, the planet, or the animals we ate. I just trusted in the systems that provided our lifestyle.

This trust was challenged in the early seventies, when I entered my late teen years; I started questioning almost everything! Although cell phones, personal computers, and the Internet were not yet invented, we had television (a few channels), radio, books, newspapers, magazines, and music. Amplifying the peace and anti-establishment movements, music was the revolutionary voice of the youth. I was fascinated by the songs of the times—from albums from events such as Woodstock (the massive 1969 communal event with drugs, hippies, and rock 'n' roll). I loved artists such as Bob Dylan, The Beatles, The Who, Led Zeppelin, and The Rolling Stones. I distinctly remember the ubiquitous demand for peace echoing through the music of this generation, and I remember simultaneously wondering why there wasn't peace in the world when everyone wanted it.

As my personal quest for peace deepened, in 1971, at sixteen years old, I learned meditation and read whatever I could find about spirituality among limited sources, including the riveting book *Be Here Now* by Ram Dass. My inner journey led to a passionate, consuming spiritual quest. I read that eating vegetarian was important to spiritual growth, as was sleeping on the floor (which didn't last too long; subsequently, I reclaimed my bed from our dog). Going vegetarian just made sense from a general spiritual perspective, as not killing animals is obviously a kind way to live. I knew nothing about agriculture, the animals, or the environment, although environmentalists were starting to ring warning alarms that we were in trouble. Around this time, the first edition of Frances Moore Lappé's *Diet for a Small Planet* emerged—a revolutionary blueprint way ahead of its time. Lappé taught that all nutrition starts with plants and that people can live perfectly healthy lives on an exclusively plant-sourced diet.

At twenty-three years old, after seven years of eating vegetarian, I caved to social norms. Over the following decades, I returned to eating chicken and fish, but almost never cow's flesh (a.k.a. red meat). I don't remember why I refused red meat; perhaps it was health-motivated or red meat just seemed gross. I returned to eating animals as I wanted to be more connected to mainstream society. Aligning with the status quo offered the perceived benefits of security and acceptance, both correlating to survival instincts.

Fast forward to June 2014, when I joined a Facebook protest against a pig rassle—like a rodeo but with farmed pigs—being held at a church. I was horrified by how the terrified pigs were chased around a mud pit, slammed, shoved, then forcefully grabbed by a group of people, put on top of a barrel, and let go so they crashed to the ground. The pigs had to be slaughtered the next day because they couldn't go back to the farm after this event. My horror was exacerbated as this barbaric event was conducted by people following a religion that preaches love for and kindness to all. Among the posts on the Facebook protest page, I stumbled across undercover videos of animal agriculture. My entire being was shaken to the core in response to the images in these videos.

I had always striven to live life as consciously and lovingly as possible. I had always been an inner archeologist, dedicated to understanding behaviors and to contributing good things to the world and to others. I considered myself compassionate and kind. But the wisdom I had developed through meditation, inner exploration, and exposure to spirituality had not yet extended to all my actions. A significant part of my compassion and empathy remained shrouded by my acceptance of the normalized violence inherent in treating sentient beings as commodities.

After seeing the undercover videos, I charged full-speed ahead to find the truth. I researched the many issues surrounding food systems: agricultural practices, human health, food security, wildlife and resource management, the environment, and the animals—mammals, fowl, and fish—who are commodified for human use. I was well aware that when anything is mass-produced, quality is lost. I had seen too often how our food systems—largely based on mass production, profit, and efficiency—neglect consumer health and wellbeing. Therefore, it was reasonable to conclude that those managing these systems could surely not afford to care about the animals, who are commodified as units of production. I learned that widespread cruelty to farmed animals is real and inherent to these systems. I confirmed these conclusions by finding more undercover videos, reading news articles and the many accounts of people working in food production, watching documentaries and videos of vegans sharing their perspectives, and meeting people who had worked in animal agriculture, including those who had worked undercover.

Subsequently, I wholeheartedly chose to live by the tenets of veganism, founded on the non-commodification of sentient beings. I felt the end of an inner conflict that I hadn't previously acknowledged. I understood this quote by Dr. Martin Luther King, Jr.: "When we liberate others, we liberate ourselves." The world is saturated with the exploitation of humans and other creatures with whom we share the planet, as well as of the earth's resources. Vegan living encompasses our highest ideals, yet we are very imperfectly human. By default, we must accept the fact that we can only do our best with the resources available to us at a given time, while working to educate and uplift each other and help heal our broken world.

After committing to living as a vegan, I became curious about the animals I had considered "food," as I'd previously seen them only from a one-dimensional perspective—as resources for humans' benefit. I'd thought they just existed, living only in the moment, not having a subjective awareness or much of an inner life. I was fascinated when I discovered they are individuals with personalities, lives that evolve over time, and languages, social capacities, and intelligence all unique to their species.

I remember, before going vegan, seeing the quote, "Why love one but eat the other?" which bounced around my brain like a ping-pong ball. I had believed I would never want to harm anyone. If I found an insect in my home, I'd put them outside if possible. One time, a young deer hit my car then hobbled away into the woods. I was so devastated by seeing them injured, even though it wasn't my fault. Despite my compassion for animals I didn't eat, I had not considered the consequences of eating the bodies of chickens or fish, of consuming the infant food of other species (animal dairy products) or eggs from birds forced to produce hundreds more eggs than they ever would naturally.

Before going vegan, I, like many, had accepted a dumbed-down version of myself by compartmentalizing my compassion and respect for the lives of nonhumans and by accepting a programmed, limited view of the world. Mainstream society demands this compartmentalized perspective as we continue to breed billions of sentient beings into existence for the sole purpose of killing them and/or using their bodies, despite having other options. After about two months of being vegan, I realized it is unethical to turn sentient beings into commodities. Because of us, they lose their freedom—their lives and bodies are controlled and manipulated. All are slaughtered young—for food or other products, or when their usefulness declines.

While many people may not embrace veganism as a humanistic or spiritual endeavor, we still must come to terms with how we live and with the impacts of our choices. So many things done by industries that are exploitative or damaging to the earth can be out of our control. Indeed, we are dependent on the resources from these industries. We can protest and demand that industries change, but most won't unless forced to or unless change becomes more economical. Yet our food choices are always in our control, unless an unforeseen emergency occurs or we live in an area with limited access to better choices. Those of us living in areas of abundance can easily make food choices that benefit everyone, cause the least harm possible, don't destroy the environment, and support food security for those less fortunate.

Through innovation and technology, humanity dominates nature by controlling our environments to serve our needs and pleasure. For example, we build homes, drive cars, and use technological means to sustain every aspect of our lives. Although we benefit our health and wellbeing by visiting natural environments, we are the only species that does not live solely in and among nature. By contrast, all other species must live in and among nature to survive and thrive.

We are the only species that is not part of the ecosystem; in order to survive and thrive, we make our existence one of domination of and protection from nature. It is important to understand that our selfish needs cannot be justified by comparing ourselves to other species, believing, for example, that because some species are carnivorous, then we are, too—despite the fact that many species, including some of the largest land mammals, are plant eaters!

We are now at a crucial point in our evolution where our unmitigated domination of nature has destroyed so much of the planet that the sixth mass extinction is underway. We have created a climate crisis that will destroy us unless we implement dramatic, swift changes. Animal agriculture is all in all responsible for over half of all the destruction of our land, air, and seas. Transitioning to plant-sourced foods to sustain ourselves is imperative to our survival.

We can choose to engage our ingenuity and technology in ways that make us great stewards instead of great destroyers of the earth. Living in compassionate stewardship, we can help provide the best life for all with whom we must learn to share the planet, allowing them to live free, be free from human harm, have the opportunity to live out their natural lifespans, and have a natural, peaceful death. While nature can be brutal to some, that's not a license for us to cause harm.

All beings should be born to live, to experience the multifaceted aspects of life, to evolve, to learn and grow, and to love. Our love, appreciation, and respect for others have yet to reach their full capacity.

We live in a world saturated with the use and abuse of humans, other animals, and Earth's resources. However, despite residing in a very imperfect world, we can always make choices based on the most compassionate stewardship possible. I've been surprised by how many people have been living vegan for decades, and I am profoundly grateful for the foundation they established, upon which we now stand. Together, we can help lead humanity into a future where we all thrive and reach our full potential.

Living vegan encompasses our highest ideals. The massive internal overhaul that occurs from one's going vegan can result in some of the most profound spiritual, emotional, and psychological discoveries possible in human life.

Dr. Rupa Shah

Founder and Director, Circle of Health

Dr. Rupa Shah has been empowering the Indian vegan community for over a decade. She is a woman of many firsts. She independently founded India's first Global Vegan Business Expo in 2020 as well as the website *Circle of Health*, which launched India's first vegan print publication, *Compassion India*, in 2018. Dr. Shah also co-founded India's first annual vegan Ahimsa Festival in 2016 and the One Earth Festival in 2018. Moreover, she has enabled patients to reverse their lifestyle-related diseases over the past thirty-five years. As an MBBS, she speaks about the importance of holistic health around the world. Dr. Shah is the best-selling author of *Dairy Alternatives* and *What about My Calcium?*

We Are Deeply Interconnected

The body is more than its physicality, and we as humans are expansive energy systems that are connected with all life forms on Earth. Here, I dip into the ancient knowledge of India's oldest texts to demystify our real nature and point out how, as humans, we can play out our roles and thrive in a dynamic and connected universe.

Five Elements as Base

भूमिरापोऽनलो वायुः खं मनो बुद्धिरेव च।
अहङ्कार इतीयं मे भिन्ना प्रकृतिरिष्टधा।

English Translation:
Earth, water, fire, air, ether, mind, intellect, and personality—
This is the eightfold division of My Manifested Nature.
(*Bhagavat Gita*, 7.4)

The human body is made up of five elements: Ether, Air, Fire, Water, and Earth. These elements are the fundamental building blocks of creation, in various combinations making up all the living creatures on this planet. We each are not living a separate existence but are connected to all living beings, to all matter and all the elements.

Existence

Our existence is not separate—it does not end with our physical body or our skin. It continues beyond our physical body. We are both a physical entity and a spiritual being. Within every living being, including every human, there resides a spirit. We are spiritual beings having physical experiences. Also, all beings on this planet are spiritual beings having physical experiences.

Our existence continues beyond our body into the energy field of the entire creation. We are constantly exchanging energies with the rest of the universe. We live, breathe, and survive by means of these energies. We are constantly in exchange with our environment.

Environment Link

We are not just a physical body; we are also our environment, which includes all living beings, ranging from the tiniest bacteria to the biggest animals, like elephants. We are connected to all living beings on this planet. We are meant to live in harmony with all beings. If we ever decide to dominate, kill, or exploit them in any way, it has direct repercussions for our own existence as we breathe our environment. If we kill our fellow travelers or suffocate them, we are likely to feel suffocated or may also end our existence. The day we realize that our existence is deeply linked with that of all beings on this planet, we shall stop killing them. We will learn to live in harmony, to coexist and co-create and help each other evolve. If we feel threatened, they will feel threatened. If they feel stressed, we will feel stressed. If they are fearful, we will feel fear. If they feel that their survival is at risk, we will feel the same. There is no separation. There is no superiority. It is oneness in its true sense.

Microcosm–Macrocosm Link

Our body is a microcosm of this entire universe, which is the macrocosm. In our body, there is a representation of the entire creation. If there is anything missing in our body, we can always look out into the macrocosm to find a plant to heal us—to complete us.

In essence, we are also all the bacteria, viruses, parasites, fungi, animals, plants, water, earth, sun, stars, moon, and air as well. We breathe this—we *are* this.

Rules of Nature

We are part of this entire nature or creation. The day we learn this lesson, we will learn to live according to the rules of nature and find sustainability. We will have peace, harmony, and joy. Our remedies, food, clothes, cosmetics—all the products we use in our lives—can come *from* nature, not as a result of destroying nature. Everything that we may use for our survival comes from nature as a gift, in exchange for the survival of all beings.

Everything from nature returns to nature and gets recycled, but this should happen in a way that is sustainable. If we ever disturb this balance, we will find it difficult to live on this planet. If we disturb the air with pollution, we will feel suffocated. If we disturb the water with pesticides and chemicals, we will have to drink toxic water and face the consequences. If we kill the microorganisms in the earth, then the soil will lose its fertility and will stop gifting us with produce, leading us to our death. These are just a few examples of our relationship with the five elements on this planet.

Earth, Our Home, as a Temple

माता भूमिः पुत्रोऽहं पृथिव्याः।

Transliteration:

Mātā bhūmiḥ putro'haṃ pṛthivyāḥ।

English translation:

Earth is my mother, and I am her child.

(*Atharvaveda*, 12.1.12)

If we do not pay attention to this, we have nowhere else to go. There is nothing available anywhere else. This is our home, our sacred space. As much as I always say that our body is a temple within which our soul resides, the same goes for planet Earth, which is like a temple within which all living beings reside. It is our responsibility to take care of planet Earth, and all beings on it as they are all only us. We are all one. To keep our body healthy and our mind calm, and to stay emotionally centered and full of joy, we need to create an environment that is equitable for all on this earth. The day we learn this technique, we will also see joy, love, peace, harmony, and complete stability return.

Dynamic Universe

We are residing in a holistic, dynamic, living universe, which is constantly changing and evolving, learning and thriving. It is neither a linear nor static model. Our thoughts are never ours alone, nor are our emotions. They belong to all beings on this planet.

Therefore, we must treat our fellow travelers with the utmost care. *Ahimsa* or compassion is the way forward for all beings on this planet. This is the first foundation of any activity. Compassion not just in what we eat or what we wear but also in our thinking, speech, and actions.

No living being should sacrifice his or her life to become our food or a product we consume. Every action has a reaction and memory, which we call the rule of Karma. The rule of Karma never fails. It always gives results at the appropriate time. Keep this in mind.

Coexistence, Cooperation, and Co-creation

From now on, we will have to learn to live with greater awareness in everyday life. We will have to re-examine all our actions and their repercussions. We will have to be very responsible to all beings on this planet.

We will have to change our perception from "me" to "us." From "mine" to "ours." When we learn to move together as a community, more can be achieved.

जीवेषु करुणा चापिमैत्री तेषु वधीयताम्।

Transliteration:

Jīveṣu karuṇā cāpi maitrī teṣu vidhīyatām।

English Translation:

Be compassionate and friendly to all living beings.

Hindi Translation:

जीवों पर करुणा एवं मैत्री कीजिये।

Yama: Non-harming (Ahimsa)

Ahimsa, the first and highest-ranking of the *yamas* (practices), is the practice of non-harming or nonviolence. At a deeper level, *ahimsa* is less a conscious process than a natural consequence of yoga practice. As our journey unfolds, we begin to realize that all inner selves are the same Self, and we wish no harm to come to any being.[1]

Conclusion

लोकाः समस्ताः सुखिनो भवन्तु।

Let the entire world be happy!

As long as we continue to perceive ourselves as separate from all other living beings (plants, animals, bacteria, parasites, fungi, viruses) on this planet, we will continue to mistreat and even kill them. Our abuse of power will return as a death message to us. To reverse the damage, we can adopt a model of coexistence whereby we thrive together with the ecosystem. There is no other way.

Janice Stanger, PhD

Vegan Author, Speaker, Educator

Janice Stanger, PhD, is the author of *The Perfect Formula Diet,* an educator, and a nutrition and health industry expert. She specializes in busting common myths about nutrition and in presenting science-based information in an understandable and intuitive way. She has spent more than twenty years critically analyzing evidence-based findings on whole-food plant-based nutrition; she has also consulted on workplace wellness programs and published articles in business journals. Janice has a PhD in human development and aging from University of California, San Francisco and an MBA from University of California, Berkeley. She is certified in plant-based nutrition through the T. Colin Campbell Foundation and eCornell.

Adventures in Myth-Busting

Finding My Vegan Voice

"I'm not eating meat anymore," declared my thirteen-year-old daughter. Her eleven-year-old sister echoed this stance.

I was horrified and frightened. The responsibility of keeping my children healthy fell heavily on me, a single mom. Up until this moment, I had been indoctrinated in the ideology of the "Basic Four" food groups—meat, dairy, grains, and veggies/fruits. Protein, preferably from animal foods, was nutritional royalty based on everything I had been taught. Cutting out meat would doom my kids to slow growth and malnutrition, maybe even get them sick. My first response was panicked and forceful. I spent months alternately trying to lure the girls into eating meat and warning them of dire consequences if they remained vegetarian. Clearly, this tactic had no chance of working. The kids had plenty of determination, and their joint resolution became firmer every time I pushed against it. I switched gears and started studying nutrition in more depth, focused on finding a way to keep these kids as healthy as possible until they finally gave up on what I assumed was a temporary phase and moved on to more "normal" food choices.

The first thing I learned was that eating vegetarian is actually healthy—healthier than eating meat—even for children. Intrigued, I became vegetarian myself and continued to dig into nutritional studies. I read peer-reviewed published articles as well as medical and nutrition textbooks and began going to conferences and presentations on veg nutrition. I learned from science-based experts, such as Dr. T. Colin Campbell, Dr. John McDougall, and Dr. Neal Barnard, among many eloquent teachers. Each new bit of information whetted my appetite to delve deeper into the science. Soon, I figured out that everything I'd thought I knew about food and the human body was wrong. Most often, the facts were the opposite of the conventional "wisdom" I'd always believed.

My Myth-Busting Journey

I pieced together my understanding of nutrition one fact at a time. Most stunning to me was the truth I uncovered about protein. Ironically, while this macronutrient had been the focus of my concern for my daughters' health, it's the center of the biggest tangle of myths in "common knowledge" about nutrition. Here's the big-picture, science-based understanding of protein I acquired (by the way, this is general educational information and not a substitute for professional healthcare for any clinical condition):

What protein is: Proteins are chains of amino acids bound together in a specified sequence (determined by the unique genetics of the organism, with influence from environmental factors) and folded in such a way so as to fulfill their function. The proteins of all plants and animals are composed of the same twenty amino acids; there may be thousands of aminos in each protein. For adult humans, approximately eight of these aminos are essential (they must come from diet), while the others are not essential (our own bodies can make them).

Where essential aminos come from: Only plants and bacteria can make essential amino acids. This means we must get our essential aminos from plants—either directly, from eating the plants, or from eating an animal who ate plants. In other words, animal amino acids are recycled plant amino acids. There is nothing beneficial in animal proteins that cannot be obtained from plants.

Why not get our essential aminos directly from the original source, without going through the unnecessary animal middleman? Now, whenever I see a cow grazing, I want to shout to anyone nearby that the cow is eating essential amino acids. She is not making essential amino acids. Plants are the base of the food chain on our planet.

How many kinds of proteins there are: An almost infinite number, when you think about the number of ways to sequence the twenty amino acids into chains of dozens to tens of thousands of these building blocks. The human body may contain over a million different kinds of proteins. All of us have our own specific and changing "libraries" of proteins based on our unique genetics and our needs at the moment.

How much protein we need: Most vegan nutrition researchers and health professionals agree that 10 percent of calories from protein is adequate for most healthy people. Human breast milk, the ideal food to fuel development during the period when humans are growing the fastest, gets 5 percent to 8 percent of its calories from protein. One reason we need less protein than we may think is that our bodies recycle amino acids. When a protein is no longer needed or is damaged, our body takes it apart and reuses the amino acid building blocks it was made from.

What happens to protein in food after we eat it: The fact that we are each genetically unique means it's impossible for us to get our own unique proteins from any food, plant, or animal. All we can do is get the needed amino acids and then build the proteins we need from these components. Consistent with this requirement, the digestive system breaks down the proteins we eat into the individual amino acid building blocks so we can use them. Some proteins are not broken down totally, and tiny fragments of the original amino acid chain may be absorbed into the body.

Why it's dangerous to consume too much protein: Our bodies have very limited storage space for excess amino acids. Our bodies are generally able to get all the aminos we need from our diets as long as we are getting enough calories, so it would be wasteful to create large amino acid storage pools. The body must get rid of excess aminos (which result from too much protein intake). Disposal of this amino waste is a complex chemical process that momentarily floods the liver with toxic ammonia, which then is converted to less dangerous urea and excreted in urine by the kidneys. So disposing of excess protein can stress both the liver and kidneys. Among other consequences, too much protein facilitates the production of the growth hormone IGF-1, shown in numerous studies to fuel cancer growth.

This basic information about protein is not hard to find. It's in biochemistry, physiology, and nutrition science textbooks. Yet people working in the field often don't stop to consider the broad picture and what it means in terms of the foods humans should and shouldn't eat. When I talk to healthcare professionals about these basic facts and the story they tell, usually the response is something like, "Oh yes, but I have not thought about it this way before."

So many nutritional myths are interwoven together. As with the protein myth, I'm dedicated to the difficult task of disentangling and demystifying dangerous fantasies about nutrition. For example, the idea that we should consume as much protein as we can is an illustration of the overarching myth that "if a little is good, more is better." The truth is that for many nutrients, if a little is good, more is likely to be toxic excess. Taking megadoses of isolated nutrients in the form of supplements seldom leads to the same desirable outcomes as eating a variety of whole plant foods.

As another example, overreaching for protein can lead us to denigrate the value of carbohydrates as "just fuel." Nothing can be further from the truth. Diverse carbohydrate molecules, mainly glycoproteins bound to proteins and glycolipids bound to fats, play critical structural and functional roles in our bodies, as in all animals and plants. We cannot survive without these carbs bound to their partners. This can be clearly seen in the unfortunate cases of children born with a rare genetic inability to form certain glycoproteins. Such conditions are often difficult to treat and can lead to abnormalities in blood clotting, immune system functioning, and brain formation, as well as to seizures and other serious consequences, including early death.

Another overarching nutrition myth that our protein obsession fits in with is the idea that good nutrition is mostly about getting adequate amounts of a short list of individual nutrients—including certain minerals and vitamins. Certainly, it's critical to get enough (but not too much of) nutrients that are vital for life. The problem comes when we drive ourselves crazy worrying about a few minerals or vitamins, without honoring the fact that there are millions of bioactive components in food. We haven't identified most of these bioactive substances, nor do we understand how they interact with each other, our genetics, or our lifestyle.

I follow the lead of many superstar researchers and nutritionists and consume a diverse whole-food plant-based diet. Many health issues that used to plague me, such as headaches, sinus infections, depression, and excess weight, simply vanished after I switched to a vegan diet based on satiating amounts of fruit, veggies, legumes, and whole grains. My food choices also include an occasional handful of nuts or seeds and an abundance of herbs and spices. I avoid extracted oils, protein powders, and other processed foods. The transition from being vegetarian to being vegan was slow for me and my daughters; we've all now been vegan, with a strong whole-food focus, for more than two decades.

For me, the outcome of my nutritional research has been a gratifying appreciation of the amazing complexity of the human body, perfected over billions of years of life's evolution on Earth. The foundation of health is to learn as much as possible about our bodies and food, and then to respect and follow the laws of nature. I very much enjoy sharing this information and busting the nutrition myths that keep so many trapped in unhealthy eating choices.

DEREK TRESIZE

Pro Bodybuilder and Nutritionist

Derek Tresize is a four-time natural bodybuilding champion, a WNBF and NFF Pro Men's Physique Athlete, and a Nationally Qualified NPC Classic Physique Athlete. He is also an ACE Certified Personal Trainer and corrective exercise specialist, is certified in plant-based nutrition via Cornell University, and holds a Bachelor of Science in biology. Derek and his wife, Marcella Torres, PhD, are the team behind *Vegan Muscle and Fitness*, sharing training and nutrition tips, recipes, and more since 2009. Owners of Root Force Personal Training, the only plant-based personal training studio in Richmond, Virginia, the pair seeks to promote a fit and active plant-powered lifestyle and to shatter the perception that strength and athleticism can't be achieved with a plant-based diet.

NOT YOUR TYPICAL VEGAN

If you had met me in 2006, I would have been the last person you might expect to go vegan. I was a cocky college guy, spending my time lifting weights and doing martial arts, and one of my absolute favorite pastimes was deep-sea fishing. My favorite meal in the world was an extra-large, medium-rare steak, with a double helping of ice cream for dessert. I've always had a racing metabolism, so putting away huge quantities of these foods was a favorite hobby. I was a spectacle at family gatherings because of it.

Ironically, I also considered myself a health nut. I strength-trained five days a week, went for long runs, swam laps regularly, and did martial arts a few days a week. I read all the labels on the foods I bought, took tons of supplements, and had subscriptions to several health-and-fitness and bodybuilding magazines. Perhaps unsurprisingly, I thought not only that meat was okay to eat, but that it was an essential part of a healthy diet, as was dairy, for that matter. Both of my father's parents had died of heart disease, and both of my mother's parents of cancer. I was doing everything I knew how to do to stay healthy and improve my chances of avoiding those diseases.

This is probably also why I found vegetarianism so ridiculous. Why on earth would someone intentionally avoid delicious foods thought to be necessary for strength, fitness, and health? I was never outright hostile to vegetarians, but I'd be the first person to make the jokes we've all heard, such as, "Why do you only eat side dishes?" Like I said, I was the *last* guy you'd expect to go vegan.

And then I met my wife.

That summer, I was spending more and more time playing the online video game *World of Warcraft*, playing in team battles against other players for hours every day. Surprisingly, our team leader was female—and undefeated. It was love at first click! After a few months, she and I started talking on the phone, and on Valentine's Day 2007, I finally flew out from California to Virginia to meet her. Marcella was something I'd never even heard of before: a vegan. Without being pushy or judgmental, she explained to me her ethical decision to avoid all animal products, and upon hearing my questions about long-term health, she provided scientific studies to back up why meat wasn't a good choice for health. She sent me the book *The China Study*. I dove into it and was completely blown away.

At that time, I was getting my biology degree with the idea of pursuing a future in genetics or biotechnology, so I appreciated the mind-boggling quantity of scientific evidence in *The China Study*. How had I not heard of this before? It was impossible to miss the fact that every health marker for virtually every chronic disease improved or deteriorated as one's animal product intake decreased or increased. It was the food!

I decided to try thirty days of no animal products, which happened to be over Lent. I had no idea what I was doing, but I figured it out. I read labels, counted grams of protein from plants (!), and bought lots of veggie dogs and tofu for good measure. I felt great! I had some serious food cravings, especially during the first week, but I kept feeling lighter and cleaner inside my body. It's a hard feeling to describe, but I've heard those words used again and again by others making the switch. I kept my strength in the gym, my energy went up noticeably, and I lost body fat from my already lean physique. My friends thought I'd lost my mind, but I was looking at wins across the board.

The thirty days ended. All along, I'd approached this experiment with the mindset that animal foods were now like junk food—unhealthy, but something to have as a treat once in a while. So my celebratory meal was naturally my all-time favorite: a big steak, with ice cream for dessert. It tasted as great as I'd remembered, but then something new happened. Within an hour or two of finishing the meal, my stomach began to ache. It wasn't nausea per se; it just felt like I'd swallowed a bowling ball. There was something big and heavy just sitting in my guts. All night, I felt bad, tossing and turning, and it finally hit me: this wouldn't have happened with a banana! Getting meat and dairy completely out of my system for only thirty days had sensitized me, and now, those foods made me feel terrible. What other foods that people ate had that effect? Not spinach, not peanut butter, not potatoes. Something in animal products was *just different.* That was the light bulb going on in my mind. This was not the same as eating a cookie but in a separate category altogether.

I banged my head against the meat-as-an-occasional-treat wall a few more times in the following six months, but the results became more severe and the appeal of animal products grew less and less strong. My body was giving me a clear message: like it or not, I was a vegan now.

Flashing forward to 2010, I was now the director of personal training at Gold's Gym here in Richmond, Virginia, preaching the health benefits of a whole-food plant-based diet to often dubious members and clients, and with outstanding results. Eating a diet primarily focused on fruits, vegetables, whole grains, and beans didn't work just for me, it was working for everyone! In fact, Gold's has a national body transformation competition each year with local and national winners in ten age/gender categories, and for the third year running, more of my clients were winning the local contest than the clients of *all* the other trainers combined. My secret? Lots of beans and greens, no animal products, and intense workouts.

A year later, I started entering natural bodybuilding contests in Virginia, Washington, Texas, and New York, regularly finishing in the top three places. By 2014, I had earned a Pro Card, and by 2017, I had earned another and had four first-place finishes. The bottom line was: *the plants work.*

It's pretty easy to see from all this why I feel such a strong desire to share this information as widely as possible. A plant-based diet isn't beneficial only for cardiac patients or patients of other diseases and conditions. It's beneficial for *everyone*. What's more, if you want to lose fat, build muscle, and have more energy, a plant-based diet is incredibly effective. Entering bodybuilding competitions, I was originally very nervous about my chances of success in such a meat-heavy sport. But after seeing success with both myself and my clients, I've come to think of a plant-based diet not as a liability but as an asset. I've routinely seen bodybuilding clients and teammates have a much easier time dieting and getting lean than their meat-eating counterparts, without all the fatigue, food cravings, and mood swings. Over the years, reactions from my fellow competitors have ranged from shock and doubt to admiration and curiosity, and as the years have passed, I've come to see much more of the latter than the former. The admiration and curiosity are what convinced me to compete in bodybuilding in the first place. I've found that just by looking muscular and fit and wearing a vegan T-shirt, you can have a huge impact on everyone around you without ever saying a word. In my mind, it's one of the best forms of activism because there is zero judgment and confrontation. All you do is live your life and lead by positive example.

Over time, my wife and I have built our lives around being plant-based role models. We now own Richmond's only plant-based gym, Root Force Personal Training, and we travel to speak and lead classes at such events as Vegan Summerfest, the Holistic Holiday at Sea vegan cruise, and many local and regional events. I've also been featured in many podcasts, magazine articles, and the documentary *Eating You Alive*. For us, there is no more important message to share with the world than that of the plant-based lifestyle.

In fact, if I had to choose a single strategy for improving health and physique and reducing one's risk of chronic disease, it would be to follow a whole-food plant-based diet, hands down. There's none more effective or more scientifically validated that I've seen. And there's no single strategy more effective at combatting climate change, animal mistreatment, and global food scarcity. *The plants really do work.*

If you are considering a plant-based diet and haven't given it a shot yet, don't wait! I've seen results that range from mild to dramatic, but always positive. You can take it slowly or try an overnight switch like I did. No matter what, increasing your intake of whole plant foods is a step in the right direction for you and the rest of us, too.

LARRY WEISS

Animal Law Attorney

Larry Weiss is a retired attorney with a BA from the University of Chicago and a law degree from the University of California at Berkeley. He practiced law in California for thirty-six years, first as a criminal defense attorney and then in the field of animal law. Larry specialized in the defense of animal activists. He believes that the exploitation of animals is a branch of the pervasive tree of dominance that exists within our society. He says, "If we create a culture of true respect and compassion toward animals, then this will change everything."

VEGAN

i embrace in my food and posture
a growing thing
a flame at the beginning
i create this day in harmony
each moment a spiral
plunging and rising in
the slow meditation of birth

having said this
i look at my plate of greens
like the earth in its innocence
and wonder how i came to this
place late in life after eating animals
whose names I cannot remember

why the silent streams
and antlers on walls
instead of deer leaping over sagebrush
to cool water in twisting arroyos?

i did all of this
i apologize to the tiny ant
following trails that have existed
since the beginning
and i apologize to jeweled insects
with antennae that feel the spring bud

but now i see the gentle cows
with their soft eyes
and pigs rubbing against me
with love like trees
whose lifting branches speak of peace
in sap and leaf

we can't understand it
but we can be it
and somehow less afraid
i struggle with my small self
to cry out and then act
for god has no hands but these
and it is not a fork in the road
but the fork in my hands
that points the way
to a caring world
it is our own souls we are destroying

i was an attorney
for those who freed animals

from laboratories and factory farms
hidden behind barbed wire
souls afire
they stood for something larger than themselves
and did not move aside as huge tractors approached
cutting trees for freeways
and leaving only stumps for owls and insects

for eighteen years i sat in court next to twenty-year-olds
going to jail and knowing that the harsh, artificial lighting
they saw in slaughterhouses would soon be their own reality
along with the metallic sounds of gates slamming
long months ahead
different from all that went before
this is what we do to our heroes
advocates for all living things

as court procedures drone on and on
they are visualizing chickens
gone, unheralded, from the killing floor
crowded together in tiny cages
who never had a chance to peck in the soil
or feel the sun
they give the pigs names
and wonder if they
can do six months of hell
and come out themselves?

they could be in an office
or safe at home
instead of going to jail
loved ones tried to dissuade them from this path
a dozen times
half remembered shadows
all were necessary to this moment
the last temptation of Christ

there is a place
where we see each other face to face
no attempt to distance or edit
and there is inexhaustible power
in this vision of all species thriving together
a spiral journey that begins on my plate
and leads to peace of mind, body and spirit
so rejoice in nonviolence
and the yoga of geese

SECTION FIVE
The Arts

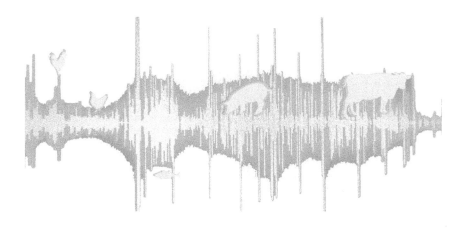

JEFF ADAMS

Producer, Videographer, Musician

Jeff Adams has given himself to a lifelong passion for helping others. Adams was a former Mental Health Counselor for fifteen years. He has been vegan since 2011 and is the founder of VeganLinked.com. Adams has produced hundreds of videos related to veganism with millions of views through two growing channels, YouTube.com/VeganLinked and YouTube.com/neofilm. He was also editor and co-producer of the documentary *Countdown to Year Zero*. Adams has made it his life's mission to help others realize their utmost potential through veganism.

AN EVOLVING VOICE

As a curious kid growing up in Van Nuys, California in the seventies and eighties, I spent some of my earlier days outside, collecting red ants, roaming to find something to shoot with my BB gun, chased by the neighbor's bully of a kid, skateboarding, and hanging out with my diverse friends. However, the highlight of my childhood was hiking and exploring wildlife. And, counterintuitive perhaps to growing up in Los Angeles County, animals became a most significant part of my childhood, teaching me about life and death.

Most of the wildlife seemed to be pushed out of the valley and residential areas into the Malibu Canyons where my Aunt Jenny and I would hike. I would catch garter snakes, blue belly lizards, orange skinks, alligator lizards, and frogs. I often brought these back to our home in the valley and set them free in our small backyard. We also raised lovebirds and cockatiels. My first best friend was a lovebird I called Squeek.

My friend David and I were very competitive with our BB guns. We shot at birds a few times. I remember one of us hitting a crow and injuring it. I worried about it but thought it seemed tough enough to pull through. Then, one day, we killed a couple of birds and hung them on my swing set. Morbid, I know now, but for whatever reason we just didn't know any better at the time. Afterward, I recall looking at the dead birds hanging there and being shocked and confused at what we had done. I didn't begin to really connect emotionally with death, though, until one day when I was playing with my lizards in my backyard. I had built a tunnel out of blocks and bricks for a blue belly lizard to run through. The tunnel collapsed and crushed his head. I was devastated. It seemed like the first time I really cried over anything, and more than forty years later it's still a vivid memory.

In addition to having lizards and birds, we acquired a male and female pair of mallard ducks. These ducks really loved each other and I loved watching them hang out. They were so beautiful and perfect together. Their love and care for each other brought so much joy to my life. But one weekend the female mallard was attacked and killed when we were gone. The male called all night for the female. So the next morning we had to relocate the male duck to a local pond. We also had pet chickens that I became attached to. My experience with these animals taught me more about life than anything else growing up.

But I didn't make a meaningful connection between my animal friends and the ones on my plate until much later in life. When I was growing up there didn't appear to be any true understanding of what was healthy, much less compassionate or sustainable. It only seemed logical that meat, eggs, and dairy were necessary; after all, it was what everyone else was eating. And it was promoted on TV: "Milk, it does a body good" and "Where's the beef?" Culturally it was accepted and expected. And if you were eating steak it was assumed you were well-off.

For me, giving up the consumption of animals didn't happen overnight. One of my earliest and most vivid memories was the gag reflex I experienced as a young child every time my father would force me to eat liver. This was torture; it seemed impossible to swallow. I begged in tears not to eat it. Later, as a teenager I heard on the radio that mealworms were used in hamburger meat at a particular fast food chain. That was enough to make me not want to eat red meat for a very long time. And my first few years in college I ate way too much chicken to the point I just couldn't stomach it anymore. It was around that time, in the early to mid-nineties, that I decided to mostly eat fish, salads, bean burritos, and black bean burgers.

I graduated from college in 1997 with a degree in psychology and worked in human services for fifteen years. Freelancing for over a dozen different agencies as a mental health professional, I found that none of these agencies, affiliated agencies, or treatment teams did anything to encourage healthy eating. I was always faced with opposition anytime I suggested healthier options. I grew more and more appalled by the indifference. I believed that ignoring nutrition was a disservice to the people we were serving. But I was alone. The stress of not having like-minded people to work with chronically bothered me. That, coupled with limited options, a hostile working environment, bills, and trying to get my family established, were easy excuses for my suffering diet. And I was starting to get fat!

Then, in 2011, my doctor told me I needed to eat leaner meats to lower my cholesterol. I wondered, *What if I just don't eat meat at all?* That was also the year my wife, Sarah, made me watch Gary Yourofsky's "Best Speech You Will Ever Hear." Suddenly, I realized the true horrors behind animal agriculture. And, I thought, *If Gary, this fit, healthy, brilliant and articulate man, can be vegan, so can I!* All these life experiences primed me for veganism. And Gary's speech was ultimately what made me want to give up exploiting animals for good. My wife and I were now vegan! It took me thirty-seven years to become vegan. Thirty-seven years to shake off the cultural conditioning, break down the dissonance, realize the reality of it all, break through the conformity, and embrace the awesome integrity of veganism. And I was just getting started.

Being vegan in 2011 seemed impossible in Shelby, North Carolina, home of the "Liver Mush Festival." My first six years as a vegan I didn't know what was best to eat, only what *not* to eat. And going out to eat was the worst. It seemed like no one knew what "vegan" meant. And restaurants invariably would get my order wrong by still including meat, eggs, or dairy. Visiting family and friends wasn't easy, either. Watching them brag about the cooked flesh they consumed, despite all I shared and role-modeled, seemed impossible. Eventually, holidays were spent either alone or with our vegan friends, who were few and far away.

But I was starting to see the undeniable health benefits of going vegan. In mid-2016 I had a physical to save money on my insurance. When I got the results I compared my pre-vegan cholesterol to my five-year vegan blood and the difference was astounding. My total cholesterol had dropped from 168 to 121. I also lost all my visceral fat with no effort beyond being vegan, and even mostly a junk-food vegan at that. Gradually, I became more and more educated about plant-based nutrition, listening to various plant-based doctors on YouTube. Dr. Greger's NutritionFacts.org became an invaluable source of information and inspiration, and my all-time favorite tool became Greger's "Daily Dozen" app. After being vegan for six years I finally knew what to eat! The more I looked, the more I discovered an endlessly-long list of the most educated, articulate, experienced doctors of all types advocating plant-based diets. Furthermore, they had been making significant contributions to science and helping their patients for generations! Suddenly, it occurred to me that there was overwhelming evidence to support *not* eating animals or their secretions. And that many, if not all, of the top fourteen causes of chronic disease and death could be significantly attributed to eating animals and other processed foods.

Would my friends and family still want to eat animals if they knew it wasn't necessary? Even if consuming animals was likely more harmful compared to healthier plant-based whole food options? I had to let others know that animal-based foods might not be necessary and that they might live healthier and even longer by eating plant-based. Plus, these sentient animals wanted to live, as do we. There was no reason to have animals forced into existence only to be tortured and slaughtered for mere taste. My predilection for helping others became fueled by my discoveries. It was now my life mission to get this message out.

I now knew that I had to apply my video production skills to help accelerate the vegan movement. Animal agriculture had maintained leverage over mainstream media for far too long. And some of these vegan businesses in the rural south needed all the help they could get. So I offered my services free to them and developed VeganLinked as a way to organize my efforts and potentially monetize my work to sustain it. I terminated all nonvegan work. I started producing content for every vegan thing I could find. I covered festivals, businesses, individual stories, and presentations by eminent social media influencers and world-renowned vegan doctors. I turned VeganLinked.com into a directory website. The YouTube channel started to grow fast. I found myself capturing some of the most famous doctors, like Dr. Greger, Dr. Garth Davis, the Esselstyns, Dr. Mills, Dr. Stancic, Dr. Tim Radak, and the Physicians Committee for Responsible Medicine. Collectively, these videos have received millions of views.

But it was through working on a documentary project with Jane Velez-Mitchell that my skills as a videographer took on a deeper and broader purpose, with the possibility to reach an even wider audience for the vegan message. Jane had been trying to make a documentary about Dr. Sailesh Rao's desire to achieve a vegan world by 2026. She wanted me to pick up on videographing where possible and edit the entire documentary with her direction. In early 2019 we finished and released *Countdown to Year Zero* on Amazon Prime and VeganLinked.com.

Working on *Countdown to Year Zero* opened my eyes to the detrimental impact animal agriculture has on the environment. I became more aware than ever of the cruelties inherent in animal agriculture. Furthermore, it opened my eyes to the incredible advocacy efforts by so many people around the world.

These are just some of the ways I have grown as a vegan. I have dedicated the rest of my life, unique skills, and voice toward doing all I can to help the movement grow. I know I will continue to learn and be a better advocate. It's not easy changing the world. But I have faith that our integrity, pure intentions, strong hearts, and clear vision will prevail.

People often ask, "How long have you been vegan?" I used to say, "Since 2011." But the journey has really been my whole life. First, I had to become sensitized to what my culture desensitized me to. As a child I loved animals. I aspired to make sense of a world that was forcing me to be something I really didn't want to be. As I became more educated and my desire to consume animals waned, my love for various plant-based foods expanded. 2011 was when I first began to identify and embrace veganism. Since becoming vegan I have continued to learn more about the nutritional advantages and the devastating impact animal agriculture has on the environment, and that most (if not all) zoonotic infectious diseases like COVID-19 come from our dysfunctional relationship with the animal kingdom.

As I became more aware of how damaging animal agriculture is to health and the environment, I also grew more emotionally attached to the animals and their suffering. The ethics are inescapable. The fact is that trillions of terrestrial and aquatic animals are being needlessly slaughtered every year. Even when I was unsure about the health benefits of not eating animals and their secretions, I still wanted to avoid being part of the torture and slaughter of these precious animals. I was ready to die prematurely if that's what it took to abstain from eating another animal. The beauty and peace of being vegan far outweighs the fear of my own death. Knowing that I spared so many lives gives me more peace with death than anything else I can imagine. Furthermore, I am now so far removed from eating animals and sensitized to it, that the mere thought of eating an animal is almost no different to me than eating a person.

Throughout my journeys I have met hundreds of vegans. Every one of them has been a unique treasure to this world. Each vegan individually came into and is standing for veganism from their own unique positions and perspectives. Some vegans advocate that the best way to start is by going strictly vegan, while others promote a more gradual approach. Some push health while others claim ethics is the strongest motivator. Some call it "plant-based" while others maintain the more comprehensive word "vegan." Some are whole food plant-based while others are junk-food vegans. Some say it's a lifestyle while others say it's more than that. Some discourage buying from companies that aren't vegan and others say going vegan-friendly is the way for companies to change. Some are anti-vaxxers while others aren't. Some give everything to the movement while others drive to make a profit and use that profit to advance the movement. Some are anti-oppression vegans while others say veganism encompasses *all* Earthlings including all humans, and then there are those who say it's only about non-human animals. And some dedicate themselves to making change through laws while others work to change people on an individual level. In sum, it takes approaching the world from every angle possible.

In my own advocacy, though, while I try not to discourage others from taking a moderate approach, I make it clear that the physical and mental benefits of going *completely* vegan are the most rewarding. Evidence has shown that people are more likely to adhere to strict veganism, especially plant-based whole-food veganism, presumably because of its rewarding health benefits. If they go fully vegan, their tastes will adjust, their health will most likely improve, with clinical guidance they may be able to get off all or most of their medications, and if they're overweight or obese they will usually shed off the pounds quickly, easily, and in the healthiest way.

Certainly, eating animals *was* necessary throughout many parts of human evolution in order to survive. And it may still be necessary for some in remote areas who may have limited options. But for the overwhelming majority of people it is no longer necessary. People don't like change. But the side effects of our rapidly growing population coupled with a continued neglect for our kindred beings is the most deadly and destructive thing humans have ever done. We may even kill more animals in one month than the number of humans who have ever died.

Our vegan voices are so desperately needed for the precious, exploited, tortured, and the voiceless. No matter how different we may be, it seems that all vegans are driven by the same undercurrent of dreams, to see this world become a vegan world. And when we achieve a vegan world the word "vegan" will no longer need to exist. We will no longer be fostering a violent culture where we are raised to discriminate one life as being less worthy than another. We will have advanced to the point of being completely sustainable even with our ever-growing population. As I evolve into my most actualized vegan self, I learn to be more in tune with all life. Being vegan and helping others achieve this have become the most meaningful and rewarding things I have ever done. My passion and dedication continue to grow with each passing year. As so many of my fellow vegans will say, "Namaste."

ALLISON ARGO

Emmy Award-Winning Filmmaker and Advocate for Nonhuman Animals

Allison Argo is a six-time national Emmy-winning filmmaker and noted animal advocate. Her films, all broadcast by **PBS** and National Geographic, have reached audiences worldwide and have won over eighty awards internationally, including five Genesis Awards from the Humane Society. She is known for her emotionally charged filmmaking—particularly her intimate portrayal of endangered and abused animals. Whether raising awareness about exploited apes, displaced elephants, or marginalized humans, Allison strives to inspire compassion for all living beings. *The Last Pig* continues her mission to speak out for the silenced and to help repair the disconnect between humans and what we consume.

THE INVISIBLE LINE

It was winter when the yowling began. The mournful, desperate howls continued for days. And then, one morning, they stopped. We'd looked everywhere: cupboards and closets, garage, basement. My three-year-old brain didn't grasp what was taking place until, weeks later, I unlatched the shed. There lay our cat, stiff and lifeless. I remember feeling sick.

In recent years, I've begun to wonder—where does our sense of morality come from? Does it start with tiny fragments you glimpsed as an infant? Or a childhood moment when you discovered that your cat, now rigid with death, had been trapped in the shed? Is it the day your family dog disappeared and you wondered if someone, somewhere, was feeding him? Or the moment when your father hit your mother while you hid behind the couch?

Do we stumble upon our moral beliefs when we ourselves cross some invisible line? On sleepless nights, these moments of transgression can stalk us: Why didn't we take care of our dog when we moved to the city? Why didn't we look for the cat in the shed when we heard her yowling? Why wasn't I friendly to the new girl in class?

A sense of shame begins to smolder, flickering at night when you're trying to sleep. It may go unnoticed by others, but to you, it is deep and dark and unforgivable. It becomes a private mark on your conscience and carves a notch on your moral compass.

Dad hits Mom and you think: *That's not good. It's not* right *to hit someone.* And then, as time passes, you begin to imagine that "someone" may be a classmate or your childhood dog or the horse standing bored and alone in a stall. "Someone" may be your cat trapped in the shed, or a lone gorilla, caged and pacing in a zoo.

These experiences are like etchings on your conscience—moral dog tags that identify who you are as you move through life. As a child, you watch, you wonder, you ask questions, and you eat what is served on your plate. Then one day, when you're much older, you learn what is in a hot dog. The needle on your moral compass flutters. Perhaps it's a video clip you watch or a paragraph you read that makes you stop and think, *I will not be a part of that.* It inspires you to shop for cage-free eggs. You feel at peace. . . . And then, months later, you see a photo of "cage-free" birds—thousands of them in a filthy, windowless warehouse, with hardly the space to turn around and only excrement or dead and dying comrades to scratch at. The needle on your moral compass moves again. With each new encounter, your eyes open wider. And when—if—you look back, you wonder why it's taken so long.

I began making films when I opened my eyes to gorillas. I'm sure, as a youngster, I saw one at a zoo. I imagine I was impressed by his size and family resemblance, but my impressions faded. Then, twenty years later, I heard there was a gorilla living alone in a shopping mall in Washington State. Something inside me stirred, that same sense of queasiness I felt when I crossed my invisible line. It was the late eighties, and it was perfectly legal in the US to keep an endangered, highly social animal in solitary confinement. Was that *right*?

His name was Ivan, and his home was the B&I Shopping Center in Tacoma, Washington. Ivan lived in a far corner of this tacky, low-end variety store, just behind the sporting goods. For over twenty-five years, his domain had been a concrete box, with a plate-glass window, attached to an off-display cage that looked like a circus car from a train. When I first met Ivan, I was struck by his calm and friendliness. I'd been allowed to visit him when the store was closed. I quickly learned he had a penchant for blondes. He began flirting, stealing goofy glances and grabbing his toes. I fell in love.

I knew nothing about making films, but I knew that what I'd witnessed there was wrong. And I knew that Ivan and others like him needed their stories to be told. At the time, Dian Fossey was studying mountain gorillas in the wild; we were learning about their nature and behavior. Still, an entire population of gorillas was locked away in captivity, brought here and bred (mostly unsuccessfully) for our amusement, with little or no regard for their needs.

I plunged into the world of captive gorillas, collecting stories and images, and after three years on a dizzying learning curve, my first film was complete. National Geographic broadcast *The Urban Gorilla* along with a PSA we had created for a new nonprofit, The Gorilla Relocation Fund. The film generated enough outrage and funding to spring Ivan from the B&I and send him to Zoo Atlanta. He lived out the rest of his days with the sun on his silver back, grass beneath his feet, and the company of other gorillas.

Suddenly, I understood the power of film and also my newfound responsibility as a filmmaker. For the next two decades, I made films about endangered and abused animals—circus elephants, abandoned parrots, endangered amphibians, chimpanzees trapped in research labs. Each film opened my eyes and, in turn, the eyes of the audience. Sometimes, the results were hard to measure, but at other times, the stories clearly changed attitudes, inspired donations for sanctuaries, and a few times even shifted public policy.

I'm drawn to dark stories, since within these stories are the beings who suffer most deeply and who urgently need their struggles to be voiced. For me, the greatest creative challenge lies in the art of shaping even the darkest story into a watchable film. It's often hard not to cross the line of tolerance. The early versions of my films are sometimes so distressing that they're emotionally impossible to watch. Crafting a film that is watchable but still delivers the dark truth is a balancing act. Whether the protagonists are elephants, gorillas, or parrots, when telling their stories, I become immersed in their world. With every film I've made, my understanding of and compassion for others have deepened and my behavior has shifted. I emerge from the film a different person compared to when I started. I often glance back and question why my personal evolution has taken so long. But as I learn to honor and respect others, I also try to practice tolerance with and honor myself. We are all evolving, each at our own pace. The crucial thing is that we continue to evolve.

I have long wanted to speak out for animals trapped in the farming industry. Industrial farming is among the most inhumane practices (if not *the* most inhumane practice) of our species, but capturing undercover footage is not one of my skills as a filmmaker, and I find the images almost impossible to witness. When I learned of a "humane" farmer who had begun to question the ethics of farming pigs—under any conditions—I was intrigued and excited to know more. I contacted the farmer, who reluctantly agreed to meet with me and my cinematographer friend Joe Brunette. We sat behind the farmer's house for hours, and by the end of our meeting, he agreed to let us document his story. Joe and I leapt in, without any funding, and started filming that week. Nine months later, shooting was complete. It had been an emotional roller coaster carrying us through the seasons, through the demise of some pigs and the rescue of others.

The Last Pig was both heartbreaking and life-changing in a way I hadn't foreseen. In documenting the story of a farmer who takes pigs to slaughter, I'd overlooked—or perhaps turned a blind eye to—the fact that slaughter would be key to the film. But suddenly, one day, there I was on the kill floor with pigs we'd been filming for weeks. Witnessing the act of killing—of taking life from another being—impacted me in a way I find hard to describe. Any shred of innocence that had still existed in me suddenly vanished. My sense of complicity wasn't assuaged by the fact that I'd long ago stopped eating meat and no longer consumed dairy or eggs. I was part of our culture of killing. I am a member of a species that condones taking life from others in order to please the palate. Eight pigs walked into the slaughterhouse that morning, and none walked out. I walked out a different person.

Once we completed filming, editing the footage forced me to relive those months on the farm and those hours in the slaughterhouse. Every day, I would see my favorite herd of pigs frolic in the woods, back from the dead through the magic of film. At times, I could stir up some faint comfort by imagining that these images would inspire at least some viewers to take pigs off their plates. But ultimately, I had crossed my invisible line.

The process of editing was long and challenging. During the edit, my mother entered hospice. For a month, I would edit for half the day, then spend the other half soothing my mother as she crept closer to death. The following morning, I would sit down again to edit the images of healthy, young pigs who would have lived another fifteen years had their lives not been cut short. And then I would comfort my mother, who would soon celebrate her ninety-fourth birthday if she survived a bit longer.

Editing was also difficult because the story itself was hard to share in a tangible way. It was exceptionally subtle—a journey inward to the core of a human grappling with his sense of morality. I struggled to find a scene that would offer a window into the farmer's ethical impasse. And at last, I stumbled on it. He had shared a story from childhood wherein he'd witnessed a friend shoot a robin with a BB gun and watched in horror as the robin had bled to death. That childhood story captured who he had been at his core, before society and culture had reshaped his beliefs. I placed his voice recounting that story beneath a scene of him feeding the pigs he'd soon take to slaughter. The moral disconnect was haunting.

It was through the farmer's story that I began to contemplate my own journey and what had led me to this place in my life. The cat, the dog, my mother's black eye, the gorilla. . . . It is these moments in life—and how we process them—that help draw our invisible line. Through these powerful moments, we set our compass. Finding that original setting can be tricky, but I think it's worth the effort to try. It can feel like finding your way home.

THOMAS WADE JACKSON

Documentary Filmmaker and Animal Rights Activist

Thomas Wade Jackson received his master's degree from Florida State University's College of Motion Picture Arts, where his thesis film *Slow Dancin' Down the Aisles of the QuickCheck* won both the Student Academy Award and the Student Emmy Award, as well as twenty other awards and honors. He is the founder of The Compassion Project, a multimedia production company, and director of the award-winning feature-length documentary *A Prayer for Compassion* and the 2022 documentary *Compassion in Action: Bringing the Elixir Home.* Thomas is a vegan and animal rights activist; he lives in the woods of North Florida with his daughter and their cat friend Obi Wan.

VEGANGELISM AND THE GOSPEL OF SPIRITUAL ALIGNMENT

Lately, I've started calling myself a vegangelist, because I've got the Gospel. Hallelujah! I've got the Good News. As you may know, "gospel" literally means "good news." And the good news I'm preachin' is that the more you align yourself with your true compassionate nature, the better you're gonna feel, the more peace you're gonna experience, the more connection you'll feel to whatever religious or spiritual path you're on, and the greater access you'll have to your divine guidance and creativity.

Brothers and sisters, I'm here to tell you that even if you're already living a vegan lifestyle, we can all become more aligned with our true compassionate nature. Some of this has to do with self-compassion and self-care, because the more we nurture ourselves, the brighter our light shines and the more it brightens the world around us.

I haven't always been a vegangelist. I was raised a Southern Baptist and grew up eating a southern version of the Standard American Diet (SAD), full of fried chicken and pork chops, *devil*ed eggs and macaroni and cheese, as well as all the fast food and ice cream I could get my hands on. And like so many other kids eating the *SAD* diet, I suffered the sad consequences, ranging from mild asthma to severe allergies, tons of ear infections, and too many more ailments to list, all considered "normal." I wouldn't become vegan until I was in my mid-thirties, living in New York City, attending a Unity church. What really led me to a nonviolent diet was studying Unity teachings about kindness and compassion and how all life is connected, as well as starting a daily meditation practice. Yet no one at Unity or anywhere else ever suggested I become vegetarian. I'd never even heard the word "vegan." Growing up in rural South Georgia, I'd seen animals killed for food, like when my grandmother would wring the necks of her chickens, so deep down, I was aware that there were suffering and death involved in turning animals into meat. But once I started meditating every day, I began to "wake up" to the fact that I was responsible for causing that suffering by eating animals. That just didn't feel in alignment with my true compassionate nature.

So I decided to go vegetarian (which I had heard of). About a week later, I was ordering something in a deli and very proudly requesting that it be for sure vegetarian. The deli guy behind the counter said, "Vegetarian or vegan?" I asked, "Vegan? What's vegan?" It sounded like something from *Star Trek*. The deli guy, who I don't even think was vegetarian, said that it meant no animal products at all. I can remember a little voice inside saying, "If people are doing this, there must be a good reason." So I told him, "Make it vegan," and I've been vegan ever since.

It wasn't long before I started noticing that at Sunday brunch the same ministers and chaplains teaching about love and compassion for all were, for some reason, excluding the animals on our plates. But I thought, "Who am I to judge?" so I made a decision to live and let live and be a good example. And that worked for almost a decade until my daughter was born and I saw the documentary *Cowspiracy*, from which I discovered that animal agriculture is the number one destroyer of our planet. This honestly freaked me out, and I felt I had to do something, though I didn't know what. So I did what I often do when I don't know what to do—I prayed and meditated about it. And that's how the documentary *A Prayer for Compassion* (2019) was born.

In the film, I travel around the world interviewing spiritual leaders, religious leaders, and seekers about the teaching of compassion at the heart of their traditions. And it turns out (spoiler alert!) that a vegan lifestyle is in total alignment with the teachings of all of the different paths we explored. Not only that, I was pleasantly surprised to learn that many traditions, even the Judeo-Christian religion, hold up a vegan diet as the ideal.

Making the film has changed my life in so many ways, including in my activism and the ways I connect and communicate with people. In the film, Dr. Sailesh Rao, the founder of Climate Healers and one of the engineers who helped design the Internet, says that when he gives a talk, he'll ask, "Who here would ever unnecessarily hurt an innocent animal?" So far, no one has ever raised their hand. Then he says, "Congratulations—you're all vegan." And that's how I've come to feel about everyone I meet. Their true compassionate nature is vegan. Basically, a vegan is just someone who doesn't want to unnecessarily hurt an innocent sentient being. The problem is, there are still people who believe that eating animals is necessary, normal, and natural, none of which can be truly justified given the research and information available today.

In the film, Dr. Rao also says that when what we say and what we do are out of alignment, we suffer. When he said this at the 2016 Animal Rights National Conference, I remember thinking: *Wow! That's a profound thought.* But at the time, I didn't get it. It wasn't until after the journey of making the film that I came to believe it's this spiritual out-of-alignment-ness that is causing most, if not all, of the unnecessary suffering on the planet. All religious and spiritual traditions teach that along with joy, there will be suffering. But when I look around me, it feels like the majority of the suffering I see is unnecessary and caused by the choices we're making.

While producing the film, I met person after person who had healed themselves of all kinds of ailments and diseases just by changing their lifestyle and taking animal products out of their diet. I also spoke with several doctors who'd helped countless patients reverse life-threatening illnesses. At the same time, I was witnessing the almost miraculous life transformations people achieved by going vegan, while I helplessly watched as several of my family members and friends were undergoing surgeries and taking medications for conditions that seemed related to the foods they were eating. Watching the people I love suffer needlessly while meeting so many others who had healed themselves of the same ailments by taking the violence out of their diets, I came to understand that the lack of alignment between what we believe and what we do creates suffering. So now, when I speak to someone, I always know in my heart that their true compassionate nature is vegan, and if, for some reason, they're out of alignment with this, they're probably suffering in some way. Instead of feeling anger or judgment toward the choices they're making, I feel compassion for their suffering and a deep desire to help alleviate that suffering. I think my concern for people's wellbeing helps them hear what I have to say. I try to remember that I'm offering them a gift. Some people are ready to receive it, and some people aren't.

I feel like we're all connected, and because of that, we're able to communicate with anyone. But when we hold judgment or anger in our hearts, that connection is muddied, even if we don't show it, making it harder for the person to hear us. In July of 2019, I had the honor of interviewing vegan psychologist Clare Mann at the Animal Rights National Conference in Washington, DC, and she gave a more scientific explanation as to why this break in connection happens. She explained that when someone feels emotions like guilt, fear, or shame, the blood rushes to the back of their head (to the reptilian brain) and triggers the fight-or-flight response. Not only that, but because we're all so connected, it makes the blood of whomever they're speaking with rush to the back of their brain as well. Meditation and learning to be present can help us prevent this. But when it does happen, no one can truly hear or understand what the other person is trying to communicate.

This is why I believe that when we speak from a place of compassion instead of judgment, we stand a better chance of our message being heard. It also helps to remember and convey to the person we're speaking with that we've all been indoctrinated into this system of normalized violence. The sad truth of animal agriculture has been intentionally hidden from us. I was eight years vegan when I discovered that cows aren't just milk machines—they're forcefully impregnated and their babies are taken away from them on the first day of life. And because there's no use for male calves in the dairy industry and it costs money to feed them, they are either killed as babies or raised for veal.

No one's true compassionate nature is in alignment with the slaughter of innocent babies, yet we pay for someone to do exactly that every time we buy animal products. I believe that our souls know this and that, in some way, we suffer for our part in the violence.

At the 2019 Animal Rights National Conference, I heard Dr. Melanie Joy say that the difference between guilt and shame is that guilt is feeling bad for something you've done and shame is feeling bad for who you are—feeling unworthy or lacking. When she said that, I realized we live in a culture of shame. Social media, TV, and every advertisement we see are designed to make us feel incomplete or lacking without the product or service being peddled. Thus, some nonvegans may have blood rush to the back of their heads upon just discovering *we're* vegan. Learning to be present and aware when that happens can help us bring them back to a place where they can hear us. Things like leaning into them and letting them feel our genuine concern or making them laugh are ways to bring the blood back to the front of their brains.

One of my favorite quotes, often attributed to Maya Angelou, is, "I've learned that people will forget what you said, people will forget what you did, but people will never forget how you made them feel." I think it's important that we, as vegans, plant a seed, or water and fertilize seeds planted by others, and then leave the person feeling good about our encounter with them. We may be the only vegans they meet. Let them feel the love and compassion that live at the heart of veganism.

I believe there is a reason each of us is on this planet at this time. And I believe it's calling to us, that we have all the instructions and everything else we need to answer that call within us. I would like to encourage each of you to ask what you can do to make a better world for those yet to come, and then to meditate and listen carefully for that calling. We must then begin working on that calling as if the lives of our children and future generations depend on it. *Because they do.*

I have a gift. I have a gift that will change your life and bring more magic into your world. It's the gift of spiritual alignment. It's the Good News. It's the Gospel. And it's the reason I've come to call myself a vegangelist.

JO-ANNE MCARTHUR

Animal Photojournalist and Founder, We Animals Media

Jo-Anne McArthur is an award-winning photojournalist, a sought-after speaker, and the founder of We Animals Media. She has been documenting the plight of animals on all seven continents for almost two decades. She is the author of three books, *We Animals* (2014), *Captive* (2017), and *HIDDEN: Animals in the Anthropocene* (2020), and was the subject of Canadian filmmaker Liz Marshall's acclaimed documentary *The Ghosts in Our Machine.* Jo-Anne is based in Toronto, Canada, and travels many months each year to document and share the stories of animals worldwide.

THE RISE OF ANIMAL PHOTOJOURNALISM

Even when I was young, I could tell that I saw and considered animals differently from the way most people did. I was empathic and sponged up the feelings of others. *All* others. It's why I walked the neighbor's backyard-bound dog and let my pet birds out of their cages to fly around the house.

Though I didn't know it when I first picked up a camera, I was using it as a tool to access and understand the stories of others, including nonhuman animals.

I remember taking photos of a chained monkey in Ecuador in 1998, as I stood with other tourists in a semi-circle around the animal. They took photos because they thought this was funny or cute. I took photos because I felt this was the mistreatment of someone, and it needed documenting. Maybe I could do something with the photo? Maybe it could help? I remember thinking that my way of seeing the monkey was more important—to us humans and to the monkey—than the tourist photos being snapped.

I had been doing "animal photojournalism" for a long time before I officially gave it a name. When that happened in 2020, coinciding with a book on the topic that We Animals Media published called *HIDDEN: Animals in the Anthropocene*, I felt relieved, like I'd finally built myself an appropriate home. I can see that other animal photojournalists (APJs) feel that way, too, because they've begun to describe their work that way as well.

*** *** ***

There's a lot in a name. Power. Community. Credibility. Naming gives form to the ideas that have been floating, bodiless, just out of reach. Naming can even be an act of rebellion.

Many times, I've been introduced as a wildlife photographer. I don't mind, as I know it's because people are grappling to find a category in which to fit my work. Animal photojournalism, however, is a combination of a lot of genres of photography. It's conservation and wildlife photography in that it focuses on animals. It's street photography in that you are up close, catching glimpses of the quotidian. Like news photography, it is relevant and current and shapes conversations about its subject matter. It's also conflict photography in that it often takes the form of an in-depth reportage or photo essay in a space that is both dangerous to the photographers and those living there. And like war photography, those who bear witness often leave with emotional scars.

Animal photojournalism, however, is more than the sum of these parts. As APJs, we're documenting what much of the world hasn't fully accepted as being worthy as subjects. Specifically, we are looking at animals who are central to our lives and yet hidden from the public view and conscience. It emphasizes the inclusion of all animals, particularly those historically unrepresented: the animals we eat and wear, the animals used in research, and the animals we use for entertainment, for work, and in religious practice. Animal photojournalism acknowledges their beinghood and brings their stories to light. At their core, the images in this pioneering field document the broader human–animal conflict and its resultant ecosystems of suffering. I was a budding photojournalist when I realized I wanted to focus exclusively on these stories if I could. With this came the realization that I had my life's work laid out ahead of me.

* * *

The animals I photograph are all unequivocally trapped in our clutches. They are pigs in factory farms, virtually immobilized in gestation crates. They are the family of mink living in a tiny cage, cannibalizing one another from stress, all while being destined for the fashion industry. They are the millions of purpose-bred dogs, fish, and mice undergoing experimentation at every minute of every day worldwide. They are animals whom we consider disposable and ecologically insignificant. Unimportant. We call them *domesticated, units of protein, inventory, trim, veal, test subjects*—euphemisms that hide the feeling beings beneath. Whatever we name them, they are still animals who, like all of us, wish to live free from harm. APJs bear witness to their lives and, in doing so, create documents that are catalysts for change. They aim to encourage swift and necessary change on behalf of all the beings in the frame.

Human existence and nonhuman existence are intertwined, and the ethics of how we treat other sentient beings is finally being called into question globally. The animals we document are inextricably linked to so many areas of current global concern, from public and environmental health crises to zoonotic viruses.

* * *

Animal photojournalism is no longer a lonely place to be. When I started on this journey, it seemed there were just a few of us. Many weren't even professional photographers but activists with a decent camera who wanted to use it as the powerful tool it could be. These days, in response to APJs, activists, and whistleblowers exposing animal industries, powerful lobbying efforts on behalf of large corporations have ushered in what are known as "ag-gag" laws, designed to create fear and to criminalize the documentation of animal use. Personally, this fuels me more than ever.

* * *

The work is brutally hard. We put ourselves at physical and psychological risk. In common with humanitarian and conflict photographers, some of us suffer long-term psychological effects like depression and post-traumatic stress disorder as a result of bearing witness to violence and injustice against others. I don't say this to dissuade people from taking it up. Animals need as many of us as possible doing this work. It is, however, why self-care is so incredibly important. People often ask how I can bear it. I manage by balancing the gravity of the work with the knowledge that I have one precious human life to live and that I want to live it happily. I also manage by knowing that the work itself is an action, which, for me, creates momentum and catharsis. I could not do what I do if people weren't looking at the images, but they are. And so I continue.

It's so exciting to see how this new brand of photojournalism is evolving and how our work is contributing to public awareness, campaigns, and policy change globally. Animal photojournalism is a small but important piece of the puzzle when it comes to animal liberation. Once upon a time, editors said there was no room in mainstream media for these stories. Today, animal photojournalism is being discussed in academia, by journalists, in interviews and podcasts, and in the global photo community.

Animal photojournalism is groundbreaking for two reasons. First, images in this genre demand radical empathy and self-awareness. Viewers must decenter themselves and consider the world through the eyes of a different species, while holding the truth of humanity's undeniable role in the story. Second, it poses a fundamental threat to deeply embedded societal systems that continue largely unchallenged. The act of seeking out these visual stories is itself an act of resistance.

This is why animal photojournalism is an act of rebellion. Intrinsic to it is the stubborn belief that its subject matter makes it inherently important. All animals are important. We are elbowing our way into public space and into the public conscience. Until animal liberation is achieved, animal photojournalism will continue to be a tool in the fight to change the system that leaves billions of animals to suffer, hidden in plain sight.

Ryan A. Phillips

Artist, Artfully Vegan
Sanctuary Manager, Life With Pigs

Ryan A. Phillips has been doing animal rights activism full-time for nearly a decade. He has spoken to thousands of students at universities around the country while introducing them to his family members—Charlotte, Pumpkin, and Millie the pigs; Jenna the cow; and Beatrice the chicken. He loves spending time walking his animal family in Colonial Williamsburg. Ryan currently runs Life With Pigs Farm Animal Sanctuary and the Facebook page *Artfully Vegan*. In his free time, he likes hugging his animal family and having his time dominated by his very needy cow daughter, Jenna the Calf Who Lived, who demands endless hugs.

Artivism for the Animals

I have tried a little bit of every form of animal rights activism over the past ten years. I once spent 134 days in a row, usually two hours each day, holding animal rights signs on a street corner in Williamsburg, Virginia; I had cigarettes thrown at me, a man charged at me with fists up, and one person even pretended to pull a gun. Don't worry, I dodged their imaginary bullet. For a long time, I also attempted to politely share not-so-fun facts with people in grocery stores (leading to my temporary lifetime ban from Trader Joe's that was followed by an apology from the manager). But my favorite forms of activism include helping people meet the real victims of animal agriculture—while sharing their stories—and using art to promote veganism through thought-provoking illustrations. And it is my experience with using art to promote animal rights that I would like to discuss here, as well as the reasons why I think art is so powerful and important. But first, a little history of how it took me over thirty years to become an artist.

I've been using art to speak out for animal rights for a while now, but I still struggle to think of myself as an artist. I have always loved art. I could spend days at art stores, staring at the vast number of colors and shades of each color available in markers, color pencils, and paints. And I nearly veganized the minds of the entire staff at the local Michaels doing exactly that, all the while sharing the animal rights message. But my elementary school art teacher, who was friends with my grandma, once told her he was glad I did not aspire to be an artist because I would be doomed to fail. Thus began a twenty-five-year silence in my art life, though when I look back at some of my art from that time, I can see where he was coming from.

My desire to promote veganism by every means possible and as effectively as possible caused a rebirth of my desire to pick up a pencil, which eventually evolved into a digital pencil (which is far more forgiving of the late-blooming artist). I have always felt that having animals tell their own stories or making people see things through the eyes of animals is the best way to convey the vegan message. Art is perfect for this. With just a modest amount of talent, it becomes possible to take what we know to be the experiences of animals and create a visual means for nonvegans to connect to this understanding.

After hearing the brilliant art activist Sue Coe speak at the College of William and Mary and speaking with her in private afterward, I felt convinced that art is one of the most powerful vehicles for transforming the minds of those not yet able to open their eyes to the truth. Sue Coe said it far more eloquently, but essentially, it boils down to the fact that everyone can write words and express their opinions thus with little or no effort. And because it is so easy and commonplace to do exactly that, most people block out the majority of what they hear or read. On the contrary, when you make your point artistically, even people who disagree with you are far more inclined to give a little thought to your argument, because they can see the effort that you put into making it come to life. They feel a sense of duty to at least acknowledge the effort, and by the time they realize what they've walked into, the "poison" has been delivered into their systems. Their eyes are a little more open to what is happening to animals. And I have found this to be true over and over again. Artivism (using art to do activism) has this amazing way of pulling people away from their stance of resistance to new ideas. I believe much of this occurs because in attempting to analyze and understand what the artwork is saying, people accidentally walk themselves into "hearing" the message.

Often, it is hard for people to fully relate to animals because of the differences in the ways nonhuman animals express fear, pain, and even joy. But with the increase in studies of animal emotions and intelligence, we now know that the capacity of animals to feel and think is not so different from our own. Art allows me the opportunity to share the experience of a breeder pig—the emotional pain she feels seeing her babies taken from her and the physical exhaustion resulting from her repeated pregnancies. Through illustration, using subtle (or not-so-subtle) anthropomorphism, I can take something that may be a little obscure to the human eye and turn it into something much more apparent and relatable without losing the authenticity of the emotions being expressed. And this often will plant the thought in the minds of viewers that they may want to consider what animals are going through.

Some may ask, "Why not just show videos of actual animal experiences?" While those are hugely powerful tools for helping people feel empathy and compassion for animals, many people do not want to be confronted with real-life images or footage of the suffering involved in animal agriculture. But these same people are more at ease with art because art is less threatening. It feels safer to look at art depicting what happens to animals because "it's just art." In this sneaky fashion, art puts thoughts and ideas into the mind of the viewer, who then feels safe and secure in giving consideration to the animal rights message behind the artistic depiction.

Some of my most successful pieces capture the emotions we know animals to be feeling, all while giving them enough human-like qualities in how they express these emotions that people walk away fully grasping what the experience must be like for these beings. For example, a drawing of a mother pig with grief-stricken eyes, reaching her hoof out toward her baby who is being dragged away by his leg, conveys the reality that mother pigs must experience over and over again in farm settings. An illustration that has a mother cow say, "Please don't take my baby!" has a more powerful and guttural impact on a human observer than one with a simple "MOO!!!"

A more controversial but powerful means of getting the message across is to switch the victim and the victimizer. People have an intense reaction when they see the very thing they pay to have done to animals happen to humans at the hands of other species. Putting a human female in the place of a dairy cow and having cows artificially inseminate and milk her seem so repugnant. And when you add a catchphrase like, "All Our Humans Are Given Cowmane Treatment," it forces those in the audience to confront the reality that they are hypocritical for the repulsion they feel if they find the same treatment ethical when applied to an equally unwilling animal victim.

For the past few years, I have been running Life With Pigs Farm Animal Sanctuary in addition to creating my animal rights artwork for *Artfully Vegan* (which I manage with an artist who has been a huge inspiration to my art, Bri VT). This work has solidified my understanding that animals experience so many emotions parallel to what we, as humans, experience. I watch daily as they experience curiosity, happiness, confusion, excitement, and many other emotions, which, however, may not always be obvious to the untrained eye of someone not used to constantly being around farmed animals. Art allows me to take these experiences and translate them into a visually digestible medium—one that enables people to unsuspectingly ingest a dose of the vegan message while believing they are just looking at an illustration, a comic, or some other artistic form of expression. Using art, we can slowly chip away at the mental block so many people have against recognizing the suffering animals endure. This is why our slogan at *Artfully Vegan* is: "Drawing Animal Agriculture into Extinction."

FARAH SIRAJ

Vegan Musician and Speaker

Farah Siraj has a career that spans the United States, Europe, and the Middle East. She has performed at some of the world's most prestigious venues, including the United Nations, Nobel Prize hall, Kennedy Center, and Lincoln Center, among others. She represents Jordan annually on United Nations World Peace Day. Farah's musical releases include her albums *Nomad* and *Dunya*, with songs in English, Arabic, and Spanish. Her collaboration with India's A.R. Rahman, "Zariya," hit number one on the music charts in India and in the Middle East. Farah focuses on raising awareness about the consequences of war and violence; she advocates for women's rights, refugee rights, and animal rights. Farah approaches music as a medium for peace and compassion.

REFLECTIONS ON MUSIC, ANIMAL RIGHTS, AND HUMAN RIGHTS

Music has a way of inspiring us and elevating our consciousness. It moves so many around the world to take action and stand up for what they believe in. There are countless examples throughout history of musicians being at the forefront of change. The beautiful thing about music is that it takes you to a place where you have no choice but to be present, to engage, to feel, and to be vulnerable. It can change your mind. It can change your life. Throughout my life, music has been my sweet escape, my refuge. It has saved me in so many ways. Writing music allows me to go to deeper depths within myself and discover parts of myself that I never knew existed. As a performing artist, I've been lucky to travel the world and share my music with people from many different cultures and backgrounds, to experience time and again a connection that needs no translation. I often ask my audience to imagine a different world: a world without violence.

In 2005, I wrote a song to the women of Darfur, who were experiencing genocide and horrific violence. Most of the world was and has been indifferent to their suffering. My song, "lan nansaki," spoke directly to these women, saying: "We have not forgotten you. We have not forgotten your pain, suffering, and sadness. We have not forgotten your rights or your children's rights." Shortly after the recording of the song, human rights activists took my song with them and played it for the women of Darfur in the refugee camps. After hearing my song, they told the activists that they did not know the outside world even knew about what was happening to them and that they were relieved to know that others cared. In gratitude, they got on their feet and began to dance, sing, and clap. Recordings of the singing and clapping were sent back to me, and it was one of the most profound experiences of my life, both musically and personally. It showed me the power of music—how music can connect people and cross all the arbitrary borders we've created that are dividing instead of uniting us. In the United States, my song became a campaign song to raise awareness and end genocide in Darfur; it was played on radio stations across the country and even at the United Nations Security Council when legislation was passed to address the genocide in Darfur. That experience made me realize the impact of music with a message. Since then, music has been the medium through which I try to raise awareness about humanitarian causes.

It wasn't until 2013 that I began to dive into animal rights. I had always loved animals. I had thought that as a vegetarian, I was "doing my part" to save them. It wasn't until I had a conversation about veganism with my bassist and dear friend, while we were on tour in India, that my eyes were opened. He talked about wanting to be more peaceful and how veganism aligned with his morals. I realized it aligned with mine, too. I did not know how much cruelty and violence was involved not just in the meat industry but in the egg and dairy industries as well. There was so much killing in those industries, and I had no idea. I wanted to know more. I started to do some research, and soon after, it felt like my blinders had been taken off. I could no longer be a part of it. I did not want to harm anyone. Yes, *anyone.* Nonhuman animals are not somethings; they are *someones.* We would never call our cat or dog a *thing*. They are someone. In all the ways that matter, there is no difference between our companion animals and the animals we subject to horrific violence by exploiting them. I dove into researching how our exploitation of other sentient beings directly causes devastating suffering and violence, and I knew I had to go vegan. It was the only way I could align my actions with my practice of nonviolence.

Little did I know that going vegan would be one of the best decisions of my life and that my only regret would be not having done so sooner. Veganism brought me so much peace, and part of my spiritual practice became to see myself as connected with all living beings. I had seen the devastating effects of the violence humans inflict on each other and had dedicated my music to raising awareness about the consequences of war, violence, and oppression, but I hadn't realized that violence and oppression were on my plate, as well as in all my purchases that involved animal products. I had devoted myself to promoting nonviolence, and now, my world expanded beyond my species. I wanted to extend my compassion to all living beings, human *and* nonhuman. Veganism became my passion, and it changed my life.

What had started off as research for personal knowledge slowly blossomed into an insatiable thirst for learning about animal rights and the pursuit of a graduate degree. I explored the human cost of exploiting animals and eventually wrote my master's thesis on the intersection of human rights and animal rights. I would like to share some of the things I learned with you.

We often see human rights and animal rights as separate. However, there is an undeniable overarching link between them. Our exploitation of animals has consequences that affect human rights, human security, and global sustainability. We may find slaughtering an animal for their meat an unimaginable act to perform ourselves, but it is somehow "acceptable" for someone else to slaughter them *for* us to achieve the same result—their flesh on our plate. The animal is not spared any suffering by our distance from the slaughter process, but it somehow eases our conscience, as if by our not seeing the slaughter, it did not really happen. The violence involved in slaughtering animals also directly affects the workers, who suffer not only high rates of physical injury but also psychological damage that persists beyond the slaughterhouse. Through my research, I discovered that there are serious psychological problems that come with continuously seeing and taking part in violent behavior toward animals. These include anxiety, depression, PTSD, and substance abuse, among others. In addition, slaughterhouse workers are often immigrants, resettled refugees, minorities, and people of color. These workers usually have little or no education and are already living in poverty. The industry exploits them, knowing they have few options and often no choice but to continue working to stay out of financial difficulties. Slaughterhouse workers are some of the most exploited and most vulnerable people in the workforce. We pay them to kill, *literally*. And *they* have to live with that. *They* have to see the blood that we do not want to see. *They* have to take the life of an innocent sentient being. The act of killing over and over again can, among other consequences, cause irreparable damage to their psyche.

On a global scale, animal agriculture has clear detrimental effects on some of the world's most vulnerable populations. Animal exploitation, social justice, and food justice issues are all interlinked. We produce enough food in the world to feed the world's entire population, yet the United Nations estimates that 25,000 people die of starvation *every day*.[1] This means that 9.1 million people, of whom 3.65 million are children, die needlessly of starvation each year. This does not include the 821 million living in hunger. However, it does not have to be this way. Most world hunger is not caused by a scarcity of food but rather inequality and poverty, which makes it a social justice and food justice issue. The world already produces enough grain to end world hunger and feed over 11 billion people.[2] Sadly, the reality is that much of the industrially produced grain goes to feedlots instead of the almost one billion people living in hunger. We have prioritized producing and feeding livestock over feeding the hungry people of the world. In addition, we are currently dealing with a conflict-induced refugee crisis, but in the coming years, we shall start to see a climate-related refugee crisis—one due to drought and starvation. According to the United Nations, we currently have 21.5 million climate refugees.[3] Unfortunately, this number will only increase if current trends continue.

It is also important to mention that apart from its role in world hunger, deforestation, desertification, drought, the creation of ocean dead zones, and species extinction, animal agriculture, in particular factory farming, is a culprit in water pollution, with detrimental effects on communities in areas surrounding factory farms and slaughterhouses. The reality is that many people in these communities (largely minorities and people of color) fall below the poverty line, and relocation is not an option for them. They experience *environmental racism*. In these communities, residents suffer the direct consequences of living near factory farms: they are plagued by respiratory problems such as bronchitis, inflammation of the lungs, toxic dust syndrome, and asthma, and the high ammonia levels emitted can cause nausea, dizziness, eye problems, and other preventable illnesses. Other health issues can include kidney problems, nervous system disorders, fatal blue baby syndrome from elevated levels of nitrates in the water, salmonella, *E. coli,* and over forty other diseases that can be passed from animal waste to humans. Sadly, at the rate of expansion of factory farming in the United States and globally, this issue will likely only get worse, and once again, those most vulnerable will suffer the most.

Last but not least, as a woman and someone who strongly advocates for women's rights in both her personal and professional lives, I feel it is necessary to discuss women's rights within the context of animal rights and veganism. Conversely, we must address animal rights within a feminist framework, at a time when women are demanding the rights to their own bodies more than ever and the cause of feminism is at an all-time high. Eggs and dairy products are *literal results* of the exploitation of female reproductive systems. We are morally against this exploitation, but unfortunately only when it comes to our own species. However, the plain truth is that dairy involves forceful impregnation and, as does meat, murder, as the animals *all* ultimately end up in the slaughterhouse. This is where we must ask: Must feminism be exclusive to our own species? Would it not also be an extension of women's rights to extend the same rights to nonhuman females?

We *must* consider how violence against other beings affects us on an individual (perhaps unconscious) level as well as on a global level. Is it realistic to think that all the violence we inflict on other animals has no effect on our own society? Could it be that this violence somehow manifests in our own society? If we have normalized violence against other species, this must have profound implications for our own species's culture of violence. If we have normalized the separation of a nonhuman mother and her child, should we then be surprised when we find that mothers are being separated from their children in detention centers at the US border?

We are all connected. We are not immune from the cruelty we inflict on other species; it trickles into our own collective psyche.

We are, both individually and collectively, capable of change. Global change is possible and, in fact, *necessary* to create a world that chooses nonviolence over violence, compassion over exploitation, and life over death.

DR. WILL TUTTLE

Speaker, Educator, Musician, and Author,
The World Peace Diet

Dr. Will Tuttle is a former Zen monk and a vegan since 1980 with a PhD from UC Berkeley. He is the editor of *Circles of Compassion* and *Buddhism and Veganism*, author of *Your Inner Islands*, and recipient of the Courage of Conscience Award and the Empty Cages Prize. He has appeared in many radio, television, print, and online interviews, as well as documentary films including *Cowspiracy, A Prayer for Compassion, HOPE: What You Eat Matters, Vegan: Everyday Stories*, and *Animals and the Buddha*. Since 1985, Dr. Tuttle has delivered 4,000-plus live-audience presentations encouraging compassion and vegan living in all fifty US states and over fifty countries worldwide.

ZEN AND THE ART OF VEGAN LIVING

Old Zen Story
Once upon a time, a man walking in the forest was suddenly seen and chased by a tiger. The man ran to the edge of a cliff and climbed down, hanging on by a root. As he looked down, he saw another tiger appear on the ground below him. Looking up, he saw the first tiger eyeing him. He looked over and saw a clump of wild strawberries growing. With one hand, he managed to reach over and eat a few. How delicious they were!

This story symbolizes our situation: we are suspended between the twin tigers of the past and the future. The past has propelled us to this current moment, and the future awaits with any number of possible challenges and difficulties. Can we enter into the vivid experience of life itself, revealed in this present moment? As the story suggests, when we are acutely sensitized to the nature of these two tigers, our awareness of the instability of our situation and of the inestimable value of each moment can be realized, and we can more fully relish and embrace our situation, whatever it may be, with both clarity and gusto.

Zen is a tradition within Buddhism that emphasizes the importance of direct experience of the truth of being, beyond rational conceptualizations and complicated philosophical theories. As such, Zen has inspired many artists, musicians, poets, and dramatists to attempt to convey deeper spiritual, emotional, and aesthetic understandings in nonverbal ways to help awaken people from the consensus trance into which we have all been indoctrinated since our infancy.

One of the main ideas in Zen is that we become whatever we practice. If we practice cultivating mindfulness and sensitive awareness, we will develop these, and whatever seeds we plant and nurture in our thoughts, words, and deeds will bear similar fruits that will inevitably ripen into the situations and relationships that we experience in our lives. This was one of the main ideas that inspired me to write *The World Peace Diet*, in order to help both vegans and nonvegans recognize and understand the full impact of the practice of animal agriculture that underlies our culture, and how its narrative determines not just what we eat, but also the basic nature and quality of all our institutions and of our daily lives.

Being raised in a society that is, at its core, oriented around exploiting, enslaving, and killing billions of animals relentlessly and routinely for food and other products compels all of us to practice decreasing our empathy and awareness, and to develop our ability to reduce beings to mere material commodities, attenuating our affective, cognitive, and spiritual intelligence not just individually but also collectively. Because we become what we practice, we naturally teach our children the same attitudes and behaviors, and like little sponges, they soak up the nuances of our gestures and actions and replicate them. The violence and injustice of animal agriculture have thus continued to roll through hundreds of generations over the past ten thousand years. We find ourselves today at a critical juncture. With our escalating population and technology, we can no longer continue practicing and replicating this culturally ingrained habit that devastates not just ecological, cultural, and bodily health, but the landscape of our psychological, ethical, and spiritual health as well.

In my own case, though I had been raised in a non-meditative environment, eating the usual animal-sourced foods, I began gradually to question many of the basic attitudes and beliefs around and within me. As a college student, for the first time, I started exploring meditation, yoga, and spiritual teachings from a variety of contemplative traditions, including Asian ones. As a pianist, I found that my new experience with meditation and the Zen teachings of practicing moment-by-moment awareness began to influence my piano playing. I had been trained to learn and recite written music, and as a church organist, was always reading and playing music composed by other people, but I very quickly found myself yearning to just "be" at the piano and let music flow through me.

I began improvising and composing original music by allowing my mind to be in an open and meditative state, and I discovered an inspiring source of emotional and spiritual power that seemed poised to come pouring through. This new experience transformed my music and my life. Instead of trying to master the instrument and to impress people with my artistry, I felt I was beginning to see myself as serving the piano and the music, as well as the inner muse that began delivering new, heart-touching melodies, rhythms, and harmonic tapestries.

It was an intensely personal experience that frequently brought tears as well as rapture, insight, and a sense of deep connection with the earth, at times with musical forces that could only flow when the thinking apparatus was relaxed and in temporary abeyance. The incipient meditation practice was fertilizing the music, and as I gradually developed the ability to rest in awareness without thinking, I discovered that playing the piano with this non-thinking approach opened the floodgates to poignancy and inspiration in my emotional life. It seemed that it was bringing healing in many ways as well.

With time, gradually, I began playing in this way in the presence of other people and realized that they often found it to be unusually touching and inspiring as well. But for the most part, I played alone and felt myself moving into new ways of thinking about the purpose of living, and I yearned for a different set of values. It was disorienting and caused considerable conflict in some relationships, but by the time I graduated from Colby College in 1975, I had decided to leave home and a career in the newspaper-publishing business for which, as the eldest child, I had been groomed by my upbringing. Sharing my ideas and feelings with my brother Ed, I was delighted that these spiritual teachings and meditation practices also resonated with him, and he welcomed the reorientation I was feeling. We decided to embark on a pilgrimage of self-inquiry and intensive meditation and began walking from New England toward California with no money, perhaps, we thought, as the rishis in ancient India would have done.

Our walk brought us eventually to The Farm in Tennessee, a vegan and Zen-inspired commune of about nine hundred people that inspired me to become a vegetarian, and I spent the next several years living in Zen and Tibetan Buddhist meditation centers in the Southeast and then in California. After learning more about dairy and egg production, I became a vegan five years later, in 1980. Through my study and practice of both Zen meditation and vegan living, it became increasingly clear to me that veganism and spirituality are inextricably connected. Spirituality is concerned with awakening us from the delusion of essential separateness, calling on us to live in alignment with this awakening and to cultivate kindness and respect in our relations with others. Veganism is essentially a modern iteration of *ahimsa*—non-harmfulness—which is a foundational practice in virtually all authentic spiritual traditions. This seems especially true of Zen, which traditionally mandates the practice of *shojin*—refraining from animal-sourced foods and products—as integral to Zen training. *Shojin* is seen as integral to the practice of *ahimsa* and essential to successful meditation practice.

I also found that both veganism and spirituality nourish musical and artistic creativity, and vice versa. During my twenties and early thirties, as I spent thousands of hours in meditation and participated in lots of intensive retreats, my musical creativity seemed to blossom as my meditation practice deepened and as veganism and fasting helped bring about more purification of both my mind and body. Through improvisationally and meditatively playing the piano, I could feel myself becoming a conduit for a healing presence that seemed to come from the earth as a being, and this led me to feel a continually expanding kinship with animals, trees, and all of creation. Vegan living provided the foundation of joy and love that helped me go deeper in both music and meditation, further reinforcing the sense that veganism is a living, transformational force both within myself and in our culture.

All three—veganism, spirituality, and music—are rooted in practice. They all require us to cultivate a certain discipline of both body and mind and are potentially open-ended adventures into ever greater awareness, creativity, fulfillment, and liberation.

Deciding to go into a deeper exploration of Zen arts, I enrolled in a master's degree program at San Francisco State University, focusing on the Zen spirit and how it has inspired virtually every conceivable form of artistic expression, with distinctive aesthetic elements. Among these elements are *wabi* and *sabi*, the appreciation and celebration of what is old, used, weathered, common, humble, and imbued with the rich depth of experience; *yugen*, the quality of spaciousness and emptiness that allows for ambiguity and openness; *shibui,* the quality of understatement and simplicity; *datsuzoku,* freedom from habit, as well as the Zen experience of losing oneself in the immediacy and flow of this present moment, and above all, Zen's deep appreciation of the natural world and yearning for harmony with nature.

The art of vegan living is discovered and deepened through practice, and the Zen aesthetics of harmony with nature, respect for stillness, introspection, and solid reliance on self-discipline and confidence in our fundamental self-nature are valuable foundation stones for us to thrive as vegans in this nonvegan world, to effectively help share the vegan message with others. Veganism, at its core, is loving kindness to others; this is also the essence of Zen and all spiritual practice. This spirit can inspire in us creative expressions that help others make positive changes in their lives.

Following the master's degree program, I shaved my head and became a Zen Buddhist monk in a monastery in South Korea, undergoing further training and intensive meditation, and then eventually returned to California. I pursued a PhD degree at UC Berkeley, then focused on educating intuition in adults and teaching college courses in philosophy, humanities, music, and comparative religion in the San Francisco Bay Area for a number of years. I eventually traveled to the Soviet Union as part of a citizen diplomacy effort to build bridges of peace through uplifting music. I remember traveling to Leninakan in the Armenian Republic and being invited to play the piano onstage just following a rock concert, in a stadium of about five thousand people. Sitting at the piano in front of the energized young people, I was filled with a deep yearning for world peace, mutual understanding, and love, and I let music spontaneously pour through. When I finished, the stadium broke into rhythmic applause, which was remarkably inspiring to receive; with this fresh inspiration, it seemed that even more musical power came pouring through in my next piece, which was received with even more enthusiastic rhythmic applause. It sank deep into the marrow of my bones how veganism, spirituality, music, and world peace are all interconnected and mutually supportive. We are all related to each other and to all living beings, and our outer differences are to be savored and celebrated, not judged, discouraged, or exploited.

Several weeks later, in a little town in central Switzerland, I happened to play the piano for an art gallery opening that was attended by a Swiss watercolor artist named Madeleine, who had also studied Zen brush painting in Japan. Afterward, she bought one of my cassettes. After I had returned to the States, she began ordering wholesale quantities so that music stores in Switzerland could carry some of my music. I discovered she was an artist and, as I was looking for cover art for my first CD, I communicated with Madeleine, and she eventually came to San Francisco to help with the album. About a year later, we had a big vegan wedding and gave birth to our first CD. She recounted to me that from the age of five, she had been hearing a heart-touching melody within her but had never actually found it in any music. And then, to her amazement, when I played the piano at the Swiss art gallery, she instantly recognized that this was the music she had always searched for but never been able to find.

Over the past twenty-eight years now, we have traveled to all fifty states as well as to fifty countries on six continents, presenting four thousand lectures promoting vegan living, world peace, and spirituality, usually accompanied by original piano music and Madeleine's watercolor paintings to celebrate the beauty and grace of animals and our Earth. Throughout this adventure, we have been able to experience how evocative music and art help audience members to open their hearts and inner doorways, so that transformational ideas are more readily assimilated. We have seen ever more clearly how we become what we practice, and that veganism, spirituality, and the arts are rooted in the practice of daily life.

The art of vegan living, like music and spirituality, flows from practice and may look from the outside like it requires discipline, but from the inside it is simply our true nature spontaneously being expressed. The way we live our lives can help bring this Zen spirit of awareness to our world, to every moment and every relationship. The art of vegan living brings joy, healing, and abundance. These are the nourishing waters for which our thirsty world yearns. During our brief sojourn on this planet, we each have our individual and ongoing path to the inner wellsprings of our unique gifts, which we are called to discover and share.

SECTION SIX
A New Future

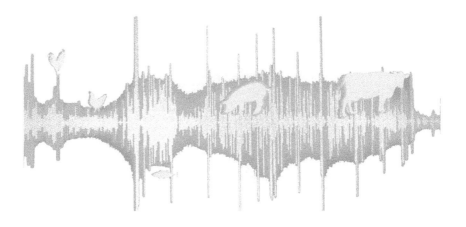

GENE BAUR

President and Co-founder, Farm Sanctuary

A pioneer in the fields of undercover investigations and farmed animal rescue, Gene Baur has visited hundreds of farms, stockyards, and slaughterhouses, documenting their deplorable conditions. His pictures and videos exposing factory farming cruelties have aired nationally and internationally, educating millions about the plight of modern farmed animals, and his rescue work has inspired an international farm sanctuary movement. Hailed as "the conscience of the food movement" by *Time* magazine, he was instrumental in passing the first US laws prohibiting inhumane animal confinement and continues working on systemic food industry reforms. His work has been covered by major media outlets including ABC, NBC, CBS, Fox, the *New York Times*, *Los Angeles Times*, and *Wall Street Journal*, among others.

IN A POST-MEAT ECONOMY, PEOPLE, NOT CORPORATIONS, THRIVE

In recent years, much has been written about the problems associated with meat. We know that industrial animal agriculture is harming the earth as well as threatening our health, our communities, and as the pandemic has painfully illustrated, our workers. A growing number of people are beginning to recognize that our wellbeing and possibly our species's survival require that we transform this harmful industry. But where do we start? How do we begin to dismantle something so deeply entrenched in our culture and economy? The truth is: a post-meat economy is already underway. It's government officials in Washington and in state and local bureaucracies who need to catch up.

Diverse interests are converging to support a plant-based food system that includes social justice activists, farmers, doctors, and multinational corporations. Fast food restaurants are adding vegan products to their menus, and supermarket dairy cases are now stocked with nondairy options. Traditional meat, dairy, and egg producers are investing in plant-based alternatives, while mission-driven innovators like Beyond Meat are producing meat-free burgers that discharge 90 percent lower greenhouse gas emissions than does beef and use 99 percent less water, 93 percent less land, and 46 percent less energy.[1] When Beyond Meat went public in 2019,[2] its stock offering was the best-performing by a major US company in nearly two decades.

Instead of confining animals in warehouses and feeding them monocrop corn and soy, farmers are pursuing opportunities to grow higher-quality plant foods for human consumption, at the same time rebuilding the soil and strengthening communities. I recently visited a former dairy in upstate New York that had transitioned to growing a diverse variety of vegetables. To sell their produce, the farmers operated a market onsite where local businesses and chefs shopped, circulating equity in the community and also creating unique culinary experiences with quality foods. Farmers are also cultivating heirloom and ancient crops, rediscovering indigenous wisdom, and rejecting the "bigger is better" refrain that has guided industrial agriculture for decades. Agriculturalists sick of being a cog in the wheel are extricating themselves from an oppressive system.

Unlike factory farms that turn away visitors and lobby for "ag-gag" laws to conceal their intolerable practices, community-oriented plant-based farms, including pick-your-own operations, welcome the public. They nurture a positive connection between farmers and consumers who are increasingly interested in how their food is produced and upset by slaughterhouse brutality. The demand for organic food is growing alongside the spread of farmers' markets, community-supported agriculture (CSA) operations, and other networks that link consumers more directly with farmers. Some producers are also using technology to reach consumers online, facilitating efficient deliveries of food from farm to table.

Despite the positive developments, however, billions in government subsidies are spent every year to underwrite factory farming. The industry's excessive reliance on public largesse was exposed in a

2018 report on US dairy farms' income that found that, in 2015, an astounding 73 percent came from government programs.[3] Even during the pandemic, most of the COVID relief funds going to farmers were to back industrial animal agriculture, perpetuating a cruel and inefficient system that is inconsistent with our nation's values and interests.

Although factory farms get the bulk of public funding, there are a few bright spots. For example, the Supplemental Nutrition Assistance Program (SNAP) has a provision that incentivizes the consumption of fresh produce by doubling the value of SNAP dollars spent on fruits and vegetables. This encourages citizens to eat healthier, and it also supports farmers who are producing nutritious foods. And in 2020, for the first time, a small number of grants went to urban agriculture to increase access to fresh food in economically distressed areas where there is a disproportionate risk of diet-induced disease. Unused lots and abandoned buildings can be transformed to grow healthy produce in neighborhoods where it's needed most, while also building equity in disenfranchised communities. Programs like these serve the public good and deserve more funding, while factory farms should be defunded.

Government resources should support plant-based agriculture, which is creating meaningful opportunities and making healthy food more widely accessible. This nascent movement can ameliorate some of our nation's greatest inequities, including those that were illuminated by COVID-19, as disease hotspots emerged in slaughterhouses and in vulnerable communities suffering from poor nutrition. Reforming our food system is critical if we want to prevent illness and strengthen the economy, and also if we care about humanity. But we can't do it alone. Government officials need to read the writing on the wall and start supporting US producers who are doing the hard work of transforming agriculture from a system of extraction and oppression into one of mutuality and resilience.

REBECCA MOORE

Founder, Institute for Animal Happiness,
Hudson Valley Vegfest
Caregiver, Cleaner of Coops, Activist, Writer, and Musician

Rebecca Moore is founder of the Institute for Animal Happiness, a chicken rescue that also creates vegan awareness and educational opportunities in the Hudson Valley of New York State, including Hudson Valley VegFest and Kingston Animalia, a "vegan arts uprising." Previous to her work with the Institute, Rebecca was active in the experimental theater and music community of New York City, where she was born, as well as a regular participant in a broad spectrum of community and social justice activism.

EVOLUTIONS AND REVOLUTIONS IN CAREGIVING

I became an animal rights activist and stopped eating animals at the age of ten. I didn't feel at the time that I was making a complex ethical decision; I had seen the frightened faces of animals on television and had met a chicken at camp one summer. I related to what I had seen in their faces and heard in their voices. There was a lot of unease and poverty in the depressed neighborhood where I grew up in 1970s New York City. I think my own state of fear and vulnerability as a child, combined with early bad experiences that cultivated a distrust of many of the adults around me, naturally propelled me to bond with nonhuman animals, whose own vulnerability and mistrust of humans were very palpable to me and completely understandable.

I never set out to start a rescue organization of any kind, but decades later, that is what happened—and not solely because of my desire to help animals and my horror at learning how they are treated (though that was how I was led to sanctuary work in the first place). I also want to see labor justice and workers' rights elevated more within the sanctuary framework. I want to see a revolution in support of caregivers and caregiving for both humans and nonhumans.

It may at first sound like an odd combination, but it is a perspective that evolved organically while I worked at multiple sanctuaries over eight years, experiencing similar patterns of mindsets and management, and parallels between human exploitation and nonhuman exploitation.

Hundreds of billions of farmed animals are killed every year, and while there is no way all can be rescued from the horrifically cruel catastrophe that is animal agriculture, sanctuaries are desperately needed for those who do make it out alive. They are spaces where survivors of animal agriculture's horrors can find safe haven and not only participate in their own healing and the formation of their communities but also profoundly influence change on their own behalf. Indeed, when well managed, sanctuaries can be incredible spaces for change, filled with healing, education, ethical consideration, connection, and personal and societal transformation. They also can—and should—serve as de facto "model communities" that provide us with a glimpse of what a more ethical and just world could look like.

Running a sanctuary is extremely challenging: there are constantly shifting demands with regards to space, equipment, maintenance, and land use issues; food and bedding costs that are massive; veterinary bills that are utterly astronomical; and community engagement and education that are critical. The high-pressure considerations associated with taking in even one new resident are many: you need virtually biohazard-level precautions because of the many illnesses from which farmed animals suffer; you have to have quarantine space, indoor and outdoor living space, with funds to cover medical care; and you have to be able to assess whether an individual can be integrated into existing groups and to provide for their social and psychological needs. You have to plan: Will we have adequate critical care accommodations for a one-ton sick cow who needs to be in isolation, or the ability to lift a seven-hundred-pound pig if they hurt their leg in a field? Is there a veterinarian in the area who even knows about and is willing to see and treat the species in residence? In snowstorms, if volunteers or staff can't travel, can we uphold care for all the residents by ourselves? If the snowplow breaks down, can I shovel the barn and coop doors open to feed everyone on my own?

The challenges can be daunting, and the staff and volunteers who do this demanding work must be kept healthy and supported. As these alternative "sanctuary communities" are established, it is crucial that, as part of the mission, the wellbeing of *all* residents and participants be considered, so that these spaces are true safe havens for both animals and people. This means solid support for the caregivers. It means creating a culture that is truly centered on caregiving.

Influenced by our society's collective experience of the COVID-19 pandemic, with a new appreciation of what an "essential worker" is and the importance of caregivers in our society, we may only hope that our social lens is widening more to include the long-standing systemic inequities and injustices that are still pervasive. The disturbing emboldening of white supremacy in this era also pushes forward the urgent need to create meaningful change. The challenge ahead is this: Can we seize this opportunity to finally address the drastic underlying disparities, institutionalized biases, and structural marginalizations that exist so that something better can arise? I hope so.

As the vegan community continues to evolve and understand its own complicity in maintaining other oppressive aspects of society, we can establish that animal caregivers can't be exploited as part of the process of helping animals. This work can take a toll both physically and psychologically. In the extreme, I have seen some workers at increased risk of self-harm. Caregiver–resident friendships are especially deep. This pure, profound bond that evolves through daily care can make sanctuary workers a highly exploitable resource, easily taken advantage of "for the cause" and pushed beyond their limits. Given the increasing number of sanctuaries popping up around the globe, it's vital for these organizations, if they are not already doing so, to adopt healthy practices that foster an environment of mindfulness, transparency, and wellbeing—for both volunteers and staff.

For me, the tipping point came when I received a phone call conveying the horrible news that a friend and co-worker had committed suicide. I had quit working at the same organization eight months earlier, but she, like many, couldn't have borne the thought of leaving—though I had begged her to—because it would mean leaving behind all of her nonhuman friends. When I got the call that she had taken her life, I felt lost. Still, I spent the next five years working at several other rescue organizations before I finally just left the field altogether (so I thought). I worked my way back to an office job and through a phase of recovery and reflection.

But something else had actually taken root and begun to grow during those years of sanctuary work, the significance of which I had not realized at the time. While at each of these jobs, I had started bringing home injured, special-needs chickens. At the time, I'd simply been responding to a need in front of me; there was no overarching plan. I didn't feel I had a special connection to any one species. . . . I loved all beings equally. I had no plan to start a sanctuary; in my mind, that was something that people with access to a lot of money, land, and resources did. I barely had rent.

I also had observed there was often a hierarchical system of importance applied to the animals, with chickens consistently relegated to the bottom. Chickens were and still are the species with the least understood and most minimized care needs. Chickens are usually rescued in large numbers, making it easy to strip them of their individuality, and often are not even given names. They are afforded the least veterinary access because—while they are treated as cheap and disposable by society at large—the veterinary establishment classifies them as "exotics" because of their different avian biology. If you can even find a veterinarian who will see chickens, often the medical care costs for them will be significantly higher.

The first chicken I brought home was Nelly, a Silkie rooster with two horribly deformed feet who had been given up at six years of age. This little guy could only stand on soft surfaces; hard ground caused too much pain as his toes were curled in the most gnarled, horrific way all around his feet.

Over the first days of his settling into the particular sanctuary where I was working at the time, I could see the staff was struggling to meet his care needs. He couldn't easily be integrated into any existing flock, and as such was left in the medical building, in a stall with nothing but a pillow to stand on, like a little island. My heart broke for him. He was suddenly away from the only home he'd ever known, in a building filled with ailing animals. My office was next door, so I put an old cat bed on my desk by my computer and popped him into it. We kept each other company each day while I worked.

My boss saw this and one day suggested I take Nelly home with me. I filled out the adoption papers the very next day, not comprehending how this spontaneous act would set the course for the rest of my life.

I remember driving home—with Nelly sitting in a basket in the passenger seat—worried about how this was going to work. But the moment he moved in, life became something magical. I utterly fell in love with caring for him. We had been needing to find each other. Every day, I awoke to his eardrum-shattering crow from a cat bed only feet from my head. Suddenly, every day began with this burst of hilarity and joy. My heart melted.

In due time, Tina—a hen found collapsed with a bloody beak on a local road—was brought into the sanctuary. She also needed special care, and I didn't hesitate to bring her home.

Next, I brought home little Larry—a chick left on someone's office desk in Manhattan—from yet another sanctuary job, because he needed round-the-clock care to survive.

And the next thing I knew, Blanche—another chicken who had come home with me from another sanctuary—was riding shotgun in the front seat of my car. These precious friends moved into my heart, and the Institute for Animal Happiness (IFAH) was born.

During this time, I met my partner, Brian, and we eventually moved into a rental that came with a nice yard. It turns out he had some serious building skills! Coop one happened, then coop two, and then coop three. By then, I had become a relative expert in chicken care and had amassed quite a bit of knowledge about the cruel practices of animal agriculture—the extremely gruesome suffering that farmed animals are forced to endure and how they are exterminated by the billions. IFAH's education and awareness programs started to emerge.

Around this time, I also finally caved to joining social media and stumbled upon the *microsanctuary movement.* A whole new world suddenly burst forth, one dedicated to empowering individuals like me. It helped me connect with others around the country and the world who were doing rescue and care work from a truly grassroots perspective— working without resources or even property, dedicating themselves to creating change within their communities, fostering deeper respect for nonhuman animals and providing them with much-needed, high-quality care, and educating their hearts out. This resonated deeply with me. I also really identified with the collective liberation consciousness that many within the microsanctuary framework promoted as part of their vegan advocacy. If we want true change and to end all oppression (of anyone), we need to represent in sanctuary structures a collective liberation stance that uplifts, values, and supports all. We must go out in solidarity with—and amplify the voices of—Black lives, Immigrants, Native people, the LGBTQ+ community, the Muslim community, those with different abilities—everybody. And we must include support for labor justice—not just at sanctuaries but for all workers (we vegans need to care about the wellbeing of those who grow and harvest the produce we eat, too).

It all started with just one chicken at a time. It seems like a miracle that we even exist, and my gratitude abounds. Every day, we are doing the vegan advocacy and rescue and care work we are so passionate about. Because of my background in the arts, we consistently bring a lot of art, music, and poetry into our outreach, something that has added a sense of joy, comfort, and empowerment to the work here.

I hope that you find *your own vegan voice* and that however you find it, you feel empowered and supported in the work you do! Your empathy, compassion, individuality, and ethics can be a force within the vegan revolution in progress—adding to the movement's authenticity and ultimate success. Never feel small or disempowered, and set your path with the knowledge that you will keep evolving and shifting course. Just know that if you keep focusing on who in your midst needs support, love, respect, and care, you will always be going in the right direction.

Here are some important resources to explore: Microsanctuary Resource Center, The Open Sanctuary Project, Food Empowerment Project, Black VegFest, VINE Sanctuary, Encompass Movement, The Care Collective, and Striving with Systems.

BRENDA A. MORRIS

Founder and CEO, Humane Investing, LLC

As a mission-driven business owner, Brenda A. Morris has spent years figuring out how to make a difference for animals using investment dollars in the most efficient way possible. After spending over a decade at a large bank/brokerage firm, Brenda founded her own fee-only practice. An ethical vegan since the early nineties, Brenda has been a coordinator for the Richmond VegFest since 2003 and an active member of the Vegetarian Society of Richmond for many years. One of her favorite hobbies is giving out samples of amazing vegan food at outreach events and watching people consider going vegan for the first time. Brenda has presented the concept of humane investing at veg fests around the country and on her favorite podcasts.

HUMANE INVESTING: CREATING A BETTER WORLD

A decade ago, any time an individual reached out to me to inquire about investing with their vegan values, I was both grateful and surprised. Grateful since we needed the financial industry to know that people did care about how their money was invested, and surprised since I had been working in finance for over a decade and had never considered how my assets were invested until a friend and mentor opened my eyes.

When Lois Angeletti, president of the Vegetarian Society of Richmond, asked me to speak on "green" investing back in 2008, I was excited to be given this opportunity, but did not yet know the slightest thing about ethical investing. I had been in the banking and brokerage world for ten years at this point, and not once had any of my conversations with clients included using their portfolios to change the world. I had also been doing vegan advocacy and outreach for years then but had never once questioned whether or not I was investing in the businesses that were contributing to animal exploitation and suffering. I began researching "vegan investing" and was surprised to find very little information available.

I did not start off planning on going into finance. I had switched my major five times in college and ended up graduating with a double major in psychology and English. After college, I had five or six "first" jobs. One of these jobs was working in the front office of a dental practice. One of our patients told me, while sweating profusely, that I should consider purchasing life insurance (he was an agent). On his recommendation, I made an appointment and, after he came to our apartment and told me the perks, signed up for a policy. I remember sharing this with my uncle—a finance guru—thinking he would be proud. Instead, he told me to "call that SOB" and cancel it immediately, as a twenty-three-year-old woman without any dependents did not need an expensive life insurance policy. As a psych and English major, I had not realized you could invest outside of a policy in a regular brokerage account. I had bought the policy partly because I had believed that this was the only way I could invest, and partly because I had felt bad for the agent.

After working at the dentist's office for a year, I took a job as a customer service representative for a national bank. I loved helping clients and ended up staying for twelve years in various capacities, getting several securities licenses as well as my Certified Financial Planner™ designation along the way. During this time, I attended a Vegetarian Society of Richmond potluck that ended up changing my life. Dr. Michael Greger was speaking, and at the end of his presentation, Lois announced that a group had formed and was planning on organizing the first Richmond Vegetarian Festival. I attended the initial planning meeting in 2003 and was so shy that I did not say a word, but instead ran home and emailed Dr. Christopher Patterson to let him know how very excited I was and that I would help in whatever way I could. I credit my seventeen years as an organizer of this wonderful event for helping to bring me out of my shell.

Five years later, in the midst of the financial crisis, I was told that if I did not generate commissions that paid out immediately (i.e., if I did not sell annuities), I would lose the job that I loved with the brokerage firm. Even though I had been doing what was in the best interest of my clients, I was let go in April 2008 for "low production." My head was still spinning when, the following week, Lois invited me to give a presentation on socially responsible investing (SRI) at one of our upcoming potlucks. I had several months to prepare and started researching everything I could find on vegan investing. While I was devastated at the time from losing my job, this failure was what gave me the motivation to start my journey into entrepreneurship and founding my own mission-based business.

I felt certain someone must have already created a portfolio for people who did not want to make money from supporting businesses that harmed animals. I discovered one financial advisory firm had created the Humane Equity Index, which excluded companies whose business practices the Best Friends Animal Society considered inhumane. The Humane Society of the US had also started a humane investing portfolio led by Chris Kerr. Jody Rasch was in the process of starting the Wide Circle Fund. Lee Coates had created a vegan superannuation fund in Australia. Lee Slonimsky was a vegan hedge fund manager whom I met up with in New York City. I reached out to a vegan advisor in Australia whom I had found and another in the UK; I even connected with PETA's Sexiest Man Alive when I read that he was a financial advisor in Massachusetts. I contacted anyone and everyone I could, and even though I met amazing pioneers who were all trying to move the needle, nothing that I found was available to retail investors. I had been vegetarian since age sixteen and vegan since age eighteen, but other than reminding my co-workers that animals were our friends, not our food, I had never seen this part of my life intersect with my job.

At the same time that I was setting up my own advisory practice, I discovered First Affirmative when I was invited to one of their BaseCamps. In the invitation, they explained that those working in SRI often felt alone in the world and that this gathering was to be a "place for climbers to rest, resupply, and resume the climb refreshed and reinvigorated." I attended this event on my way to the New York Veg Expo in Albany and was pleasantly surprised that rather than pushing products and exhausting us with sales pitches, the speakers were discussing "greening" the Empire State Building and getting BPA out of baby bottles. I was excited to find a group of people motivated by using their investment dollars for good. Steve Schueth, the president of the network at the time, was even present when Nelson Mandela thanked investors for helping to end apartheid. This group was the real deal.

At my first SRI conference with my new colleagues several months later, I was pleased to see meatless burgers offered at dinner. My initial excitement quickly diminished when I saw that at the end of the buffet line, there were also carving stations, with servers eager to cut off a slab of meat for anyone who was interested. Conference attendees, who purportedly cared very much about the environment, were interested in directing their investments in "healthy, life-affirming ways," as stated in the program brochure. Yet how could these same people also be eating animals at a conference that was otherwise so uplifting and positive?

In 2015, a friend from a mutual fund company who knew of my passion and mission told me about FAIRR, the Farm Animal Risk and Return initiative, and its founder, Jeremy Coller. I felt validated to have finally found an organization that was doing what I was determined to do, but with a lot more money and, arguably, a lot more success. While I had been asking funds to be more animal-friendly for years at this point, I now had a concrete way of asking portfolio managers to get on board. By joining FAIRR, asset managers were committing to acknowledging as part of their investment process the many risks associated with intensive livestock production.

I began encouraging portfolio managers with whom we worked to join FAIRR. One instance involved the portfolio manager of an emerging market fund, whom we had employed. Soon after he joined at my urging, I discovered a poultry producer in the portfolio he managed. I reached out immediately to let him know that I found this at odds with his being a FAIRR member, asking to hear his thoughts. After explaining that the fund's strategy was passive in nature, to his credit, he removed the holding as soon as he was able to do so. Here was an example of how mandated screens like tobacco, GMOs, gambling, and defense contractors did not automatically exclude meat producers. Shares were sold in all accounts managed by this asset manager as a result of this one interaction. I then wrote to the poultry producer's investor relations department, asking the company to move toward plant-based proteins while letting it know that our clients did not wish to invest in companies whose business models generated profit solely from the exploitation and killing of animals.

While animal advocacy groups have worked on shareholder advocacy for years now, more recently, groups like PETA have kicked up their efforts a notch with an exciting initiative to encourage traditional "meat" companies that have acquired or developed vegan alternatives to shut down slaughter lines altogether and embrace plant-based meats. My excitement turned into disappointment when I learned that one of the oldest SRI mutual fund families in the country refused to use its position in one of the businesses being targeted to support this initiative. Since our own money managers typically would not hold the worst of these companies, we were unable to assist with this engagement directly, or so I thought. I decided to participate in the investor call myself and was thrilled when the moderator requested that the CEO respond to my inquiry about embracing plant-based proteins in light of all of the many risks associated with "conventional livestock." (This particular company had acquired two other previously all-vegan companies.) Happily, the only other investor inquiry on the call came from another animal activist, and the question they posed to the CEO was also about moving toward plant-based options.

Looking back, I believe that when I started, I was providing a solution that few needed or even wanted yet. Just as I had never considered whether my own funds were doing harm or not, I discovered that many other animal advocates had also not yet made the connection. I see the folks who did contact me in their search for an advisor focused on ethical investing as more enlightened than I was. They figured this out on their own, whereas I had to have my eyes opened by Lois. A decade later, there is now a small group of vegan financial advisors in the humane investing space with whom I collaborate. For our shared mission to create a better world using investment dollars to quickly succeed, we need as many people working on it as possible.

While assisting those who are inspired to change the world is personally fulfilling, I take seriously the incredible responsibility my clients have given me as well as the trust they have placed in me. I encourage anyone who cares about animals to invest in companies that do not support, cause, or contribute to animal exploitation and suffering, although I hope this specialization is not needed much longer as more and more businesses move toward incorporating cruelty-free practices into their business models. Since most of us need to invest for the future anyhow, in the process, why not invest in companies and businesses that are at least trying to make the world a better place for all beings?

ABHAY RANGAN

Founder, Goodmylk

Abhay Rangan has been a champion for animal rights in India since the age of sixteen. After running a successful nonprofit focused on veganism throughout his teen years, he launched Goodmylk in 2016 with a mission to make affordable cruelty-free dairy alternatives. Abhay originally created each Goodmylk product with his mother in their home kitchen, but their plant-based foods now reach thousands of families across the country. Goodmylk is one of India's leading plant-based dairy companies. They create delicious, functional, and accessible dairy products made from plants, designed to replace animal-based dairy products at scale. Abhay also carries the distinction of being on the Forbes 30 Under 30 list for Asia and for India at age twenty-two.

TOOLS FOR A NEW WORLD

My journey started when I was thirteen. My parents turned vegan in 2010, and I remember choosing to do the same, along with my sister, on January 1, 2011. As I was born into a family that strove for academic and artistic excellence, there was a lot of encouragement to be ambitious and to think big. My mother recommended the book *The Magic of Thinking Big* by David J. Schwartz, and I remember reading it over and over again in eighth grade.

Naturally, my ambition came to involve doing something big for the animal rights movement. Going vegan had transformed my worldview into one based on rationality, and I began to question things I had been conditioned to believe but couldn't really find the evidence for. I started volunteering at fourteen and, at sixteen, launched my own grassroots nonprofit that focused on campaigns for animal rights awareness. When I was nineteen, Goodmylk was born as an effort to make plant-based foods accessible, and it was off to the races.

While we hold expectations that the world will eventually be vegan, speed is of the essence. More than sixty-two billion land animals and three trillion marine animals are killed every year. The longer we wait, the higher the death toll of animal agriculture and the more devastating its consequences on our planet. Our responsibility as representatives of the movement is to figure out not only the most effective strategies, but also the quickest. What I am completely drawn to is the idea of a multipronged approach—institutional, governmental, and corporate outreach on the one hand, and individual outreach on the other. Looking back, I can identify some key strategies that I believe can help catapult our movement forward.

The Power of Leverage

Leverage amplifies and creates results that are disproportionate to the effort put in. Leverage exists in multiple formats—through people, media, capital, or technology. High-growth companies in our space are a powerful nexus of different types of leverage, and having more of them helps our movement grow faster. Leverage can do more!

In our own case, Goodmylk has grown past the limitations of my intellect and ability, owing to the talent we have been able to bring on board and retain. Our people are powerhouses of knowledge and drive and have helped us solve key problems. Our capital raises have helped us reach more customers; our technology stack has helped customers find and order from us 24/7; and our story is amplified by the power of community and media houses.

Free markets allow consumers to vote with their money, and consumers who care about our movement will incentivize the custodians of leverage—banks, VC/PE (venture capital/private equity) players, fund houses, media houses, and politicians—to align themselves with the interests of our movement.

Self-Development for Changemakers

Today's most effective changemakers are well-spoken and calm, understanding of how our world works, willing to engage with all stakeholders of the system we're trying to change, and—dare I say it?—happy. Our movement is unique—we are not the victims. We are representatives and voices for the animals. It is our responsibility to be the best we can be. All the people I admire today are not only uncompromising and steadfast in their ideals but also humble, polite, accountable, and punctual.

Although there is certainly a place for all kinds of approaches, using only aggressive or angry ones ignores nuance and context. Social media has given everyone the opportunity to broadcast, and owing to the nature of its algorithms, most of what we see are outrage-seeking, virtue-signaling approaches, and these usually do not translate successfully offline. I wish for the advocates of our movement to be happy, healthy, and—yes—wealthy. Much of this can be achieved simply by focusing on being our best possible selves.

I see a version of our movement, one that is already unfolding, wherein everyone has figured out how they can be most effective, whether as lawyers, accountants, capital allocators, scientists, health professionals, politicians, educators, writers, speakers, community organizers, activists, or animal rescuers—all working together and helping each other be the best they can be. The day is not far off when our movement will see consumers spending north of a trillion dollars, political parties appealing to voters who care about animal rights, banks with significant exposure to industry, and the best of the world employed to herald a new clean, green, and lean future.

Systems-Level Thinking

The best changemakers I know are deep, systems-level thinkers. They do not see issues as standalone but as an interplay of elements—sometimes at random—leaving open opportunities for change. There is an innate understanding that we all have a place in the system and are able to influence some parts of it better than others. It is critical to develop a way of understanding "the whole picture" so we may avoid unintended consequences.

An understanding of *ikigai*—defined as the convergence of one's passion, beliefs, values, and vocation—may help us figure out where we can be the most effective and, more importantly, the most fulfilled.

Our movement has had multiple waves over time—represented by direct action, abolition, single-issue campaigns, and so on—each often led by a few compelling proponents. A good systems-level thinker knows that there is space for all of these, and a combination of approaches helps us extract the best outcomes. An important corollary is to avoid using a bad approach that we're convinced is right, as it is often better to avoid irrationality than to seek brilliance. As is the nature of compounding, our movement has started with small wins. These wins will continue to compound over time to become an avalanche. When animal rights issues have become a big part of society's consciousness and dialogue, so we may establish necessary protections for animals and move on to other problems.

We may reasonably predict—looking at some lessons from history—that a combination of factors will result in the vast majority of the world eating food that doesn't come from an animal. There will be overwhelming consumer demand, brought about by awareness-generating campaigns, changes in legislation, and other incentives. Widespread supplies of these alternative foods will eventually undercut meat, dairy, and egg prices; a combination of plant-based, fermentation, and cellular agriculture technologies will constitute a new future of food production.

Our future is an exciting one. As we turn our focus to colonizing space, eradicating disease, enabling robots to do tasks we don't want to do, solving nuclear fusion, and more, we mustn't forget the moral fabric that holds our society together. So many decisions that we make as a species will be guided by ethics. Veganism is a bold, beautiful, and powerful way to start heralding the future and to help humanity tread the path of being a rational, kind, compassionate group of individuals who champion the same ethics. No matter how many planets we conquer and inhabit, we will not escape our conscience.

DR. SAILESH RAO

Executive Director, Climate Healers

Sailesh Rao, PhD, is an author, Human Earth Animal Liberation (HEAL) activist, the executive director of Climate Healers—a nonprofit dedicated to healing the earth's climate—a husband, a dad, and since 2010, a star-struck grandfather. In 2016, he promised his granddaughter Kimaya that the world would be vegan by the time she turned sixteen, in 2026, and that people would stop eating her relatives, the animals. He has faith that humanity will transform, not just for ethical reasons but also out of sheer ecological necessity, so that he can keep his unbreakable pinky promise to Kimaya.

IMAGINEERING A VEGAN WORLD BY 2026!

We are in the midst of the greatest transformation in human history, one akin to the metamorphosis of a Caterpillar into a Butterfly. This transformation is from a predator species to a caretaker species, as we reconfigure our system of normalized violence into a system of normal nonviolence. At present, this transformation is happening one individual at a time, but as the vegan movement gathers momentum, it will inevitably snowball into the necessary systemic overhaul. Such systemic renovation requires a sea change in the stories we tell and the games we play, for that's how we humans coordinate our actions among millions and billions of us to form a civilization.

Let's begin with the true story of an individual, Paul Chatlin, from West Bloomfield, Michigan.[4] In 2013, Paul was in his early fifties, and he had a problem, a big problem. He couldn't walk ten steps without feeling excruciating chest pain. His cardiologist diagnosed that his heart was enlarged, with its right side thickened, while one of his major arteries was 100 percent blocked and two others were 65 percent blocked. He gave Paul two options for treatment:

A. Go on a plant-based vegan diet, or
B. Undergo triple bypass heart surgery.

Paul chose option A. He took a cooking course offered by Dr. Caldwell Esselstyn and Ann Esselstyn and learned how to thrive on a healthy vegan diet. It cost him $975, and his heart disease literally disappeared. Indeed, as Dr. Esselstyn and his colleagues tirelessly point out, heart disease is mostly just a case of chronic food poisoning. When the patient starts eating right, the body can heal and melt the heart disease away.

When Paul Chatlin tried to get the cost of his cooking classes reimbursed through his health insurance provider, Blue Cross/Blue Shield (BC/BS), it refused. He escalated his claim all the way up to the BC/BS headquarters, pointing out the absurdity of the company's willingness to cut a check for $125,000 for a triple bypass heart surgery, but not for $975 for cooking classes. His claim was denied, and he was told to contact his state legislators for any policy changes on this matter. You see, our healthcare system has no "code" for cooking classes. It has plenty of codes for pills and procedures to let corporations make money off our diseases, but no code for the cure.

Our global climate change/ecological predicament is akin to Paul Chatlin's personal health saga, multiplied by millions and billions of individuals. Billionaires and corporations are angling to make trillions of dollars off the "triple bypass surgeries" they are prescribing for the planet in the form of a "Green New Deal," while they have no "code" for the cure that is lifestyle change. They are still stuck in humanity's violent Caterpillar mindset, playing a finite game of economic growth with a top–down money flow, which:[5]

1) *Monetizes everything* so that when dead trees have more economic value than live trees, they bulldoze trees; when dead animals have more economic value than live animals, they slaughter animals; and

when sick humans have more economic value than healthy humans, they make people sick;

2) *Endangers life on Earth* through climate change, biological annihilation, chemical pollution, and pandemics;

3) *Addicts everyone* to compulsive behaviors in order to maximize corporate revenues and profits;

4) *Lies to us* about the basics of nutrition, the root cause of climate change and pandemics, the toxicity of industrial processes and products; and

5) *Steals from the poor* in order to enrich the rich. When we buy a pound of organic rice in the supermarket for $2, a mere $0.05 trickles down to the poor family that grew the rice in Asia, leaving the rest for wealthy corporate traders. Through such daylight robbery, corporations currently siphon an estimated $3 trillion of wealth from the global South to the global North annually.

Please note that this game is contrary to the one that Americans agreed to play over two hundred years ago. Culture is a "specification" of the game, while civilization is its engineering implementation. The American cultural ideal, as stated in the Declaration of Independence (1776), is truly lofty:

We hold these truths to be self-evident, that all men [beings] are created equal, that they are endowed by their Creator with certain unalienable Rights, that among these are Life, Liberty and the pursuit of Happiness.

Yet the American civilization is spearheading the very opposite of this ideal in the global economic game.

COVID-19 is just an overt manifestation of the global public health crisis that has been building up for centuries, mainly due to a food system that is an engineering shambles. We are extracting *six* times as much food as we really need from the planet, and yet even in this country, the richest in the world, 97 percent of Americans are not getting enough fiber in their diets; 98 percent are deficient in potassium; 68 percent are deficient in magnesium; and so on, down the list of essential minerals.[6] Indeed, the obesity epidemic in America is truly an epidemic of malnutrition. The US Department of Agriculture (USDA) is dutifully reporting these statistics, but the Food and Drug Administration (FDA) and the Centers for Disease Control (CDC) are doing little to nothing about them, because they have no "code" for the cure but plenty of codes to help corporations make money off our diseases. How can we solve our ecological public health crisis by continuing to develop and propagate this game? Will we solve it when Indians and Chinese are also as chronically diseased as Americans?

Of course, we won't.

Yet the mainstream media tells us stories about how the whole world is eager to continue playing this finite game centered on an obsession with growth. Believe me, I have spoken to the families in India that grow the organic rice, and they would rather get compensated fairly for their efforts than play this game. It is only those in the privileged class, who haven't yet realized that they are also being factory-farmed, who wish to continue this economic game.

This game is factory-farming all of us by turning us into debt slaves and privileged prisoners. The privileged build walls to isolate themselves, succumbing to alcohol and drug abuse in their isolation, while the vast majority starve or slave away at jobs to pay off their debts. Even as the COVID-19 pandemic hit, vast public resources worldwide were allocated for developing vaccines but not for helping people overcome the co-morbidities—diabetes, heart disease, lung disease, and hypertension—that make COVID-19 lethal. Now, we are being told that multiple miracle vaccines have been developed in less than a quarter of the time that every other vaccine development in the history of humankind has taken. Therefore, we can stay complacent that the Caterpillar economy can continue to grow and does not have to enter its Chrysalis phase.

Color me skeptical.

Trillions of trees, trillions of animals, and millions of humans have already died prematurely as corporations and public officials lurched from emergency to emergency, conducting the Caterpillar's violent game. But we don't have to wait until trillions more die before their time and even risk precipitating our own extinction. Like Paul Chatlin, we can collectively opt for the cure, the necessary lifestyle change that is global veganism. Besides, once we acknowledge that we humans are causing climate change, don't we have the responsibility to stabilize the earth's climate and prevent any more ice ages from ever occurring? Therein we have acquired a purpose for our continued existence—for the benefit of all Earthlings.

To coordinate our actions in a nonviolent Vegan World, we can imagine and engineer a new economic game that is closer to our ideal, one that indeed treats all beings with equal respect and guarantees the basic necessities of life so that every human being can exercise the unalienable right to life, liberty, and the pursuit of happiness. We base this new, "infinite" game, **Aquarius**, on Kate Raworth's *Doughnut Economics* to usher in the Chrysalis phase of our existence. This is a game that:[7]

1) *Monitors our ecological impact* so that humanity stays within planetary boundaries with regards to climate change, land use, fresh water use, nitrogen and phosphorous cycles, ocean acidification, chemical pollution, atmospheric aerosol loading, ozone depletion, and biodiversity loss;

2) *Enriches life on Earth* through watershed restoration, native ecosystem regeneration, and food forests;

3) *Inspires everyone* to compassionate action;

4) *Aligns with the truth* about the basics of human nutrition and the root cause of climate change and pandemics, while being transparent about the toxicity of industrial processes and products; and

5) *Serves hitherto underprivileged* humans and animals in order to restore their dignity and honor their sacrifice during the Caterpillar's violent game.

Aquarius is an infinite game because it continuously keeps us within the best known estimates of our planet's boundaries and therefore can be played forever. And best of all, we can play the *Aquarius* game in conjunction with the Caterpillar's finite game, thereby transitioning smoothly with the goal of discontinuing the finite game by 2026.

If this resonates with you, please bring your gifts and contribute to the online quarterly convergences as we work to realize a Vegan World by 2026!

STEPHANIE REDCROSS WEST

Founder, Vegan Mainstream

Inspiring vegans in business is a passion of Vegan Mainstream Founder and Managing Director Stephanie Redcross West. In 2009, after fifteen years in small business and Fortune 500 marketing, Stephanie began blazing a trail as a leader in the vegan business world. Since then, she has been building Vegan Mainstream into the invaluable resource it has become, all while collaborating with other key organizations in the vegan movement. She frequently speaks at vegan events, writes articles for vegan magazines, and participates in vegan business forums. Stephanie is constantly seeking new ways to help motivate others to move veganism forward. Recently, she has started focusing on creating innovative ways to meet the expanding needs of the vegan business community via online courses, a free business support group, and podcasting.

PURPOSEFULLY DREAMING OF A VEGAN FUTURE

I've been a dreamer all my life, and from early on, I've understood the power that dreams can have. I believe purposeful dreaming is actually an important life skill, one I practice because I want to ensure I am the architect of my own life. No one can know or control the future, but I have come to understand that there are moments in life when I will be faced with a choice or a chance to make an impactful decision. When those moments come, I always want to be ready, and purposeful dreaming helps me achieve that.

When I was five years old, I became interested in Japanese culture. While my interest had originated from some of the food I had been eating at restaurants, it slowly transformed into a passion for Japanese photography, literature, and arts. As I grew older, the idea of working and living in Japan became a dream of mine. I had the chance to realize my dream in 1995, when I spent the summer studying in Japan. Then in 2003, I went back to work there and even flew my family to Tokyo that year to celebrate Christmas. Those experiences taught me that if I could dream it, I could do it, and since then, I have made it a lifetime habit to choose a big dream every few years to work toward. Those purposeful dreams have become my guides, helping me to make decisions and consistently take actions that will enable them to become realities. This practice keeps me focused on accomplishing extraordinary things in my life.

Early in my career, I began applying this practice to my long-term career goals. At a young age, I started out with an enviable career in corporate America and was blessed with opportunities and the acquaintance of amazing people who helped guide me on the path to success. But after just a few years, I found myself wanting something more. As I reflected, I began to understand that true fulfillment would mean aligning my career with my deepest passion.

This meant I needed to find a way to make veganism a larger part of my work life, and I knew it was time to go back to the dreaming board. How could I align my vegan lifestyle with my passion for business, marketing, and community development? I began to envision a world filled with all varieties and descriptions of vegan businesses. An ethical marketplace run by people who cared just as deeply about doing good as they did about their bottom line. How could I help to create such a world?

The answer was born when I founded my company, Vegan Mainstream, in 2009.

Back then, more than twelve years ago, "vegan business" was barely a term anyone was using, let alone one that denoted a significant part of the marketplace. As I introduced Vegan Mainstream and let people know that I was here to support vegan businesses with their business and marketing needs, it quickly became clear that I represented a niche inside a niche. I loved talking about the power of vegan marketing and how we could build a vegan economy, but most veg fests and other similar venues doubted that audiences would be interested. I was a little ahead of my time, but because of my dream, I didn't give up. In it, I could see a version of the reality we are living in today. I used the training I had received from my experience in corporate America, along with my entrepreneurial family background, to study social movements, marketing trends, and business cycles. Of course, I can no more predict the future than can anyone, but by using all the skills, training, and resources at my disposal, I was able to glimpse the possibilities of my dream.

And in truth, helping others to realize the path to making their vegan business dreams come true is what Vegan Mainstream has really become about in the past decade. It's not just about sharing tools and practical, actionable business advice and know-how (important as these are), but it's also about holding space for the vision of a collective dream, one that contains a better future for animals, the planet, and humans as well.

Without a doubt, one of the most rewarding parts of my career is helping others find the light at the end of a gloomy tunnel, while letting them know that I'm willing to walk down a dark, winding road with them because I, too, can see what they see.

The world can be vegan, but we must create the right environment for that to occur. And a key part of that process is holding fast to the dream, never letting it go.

Vegan Mainstream is driven by the desire to create a mainstream vegan movement. This means ensuring that vegan options are accessible to everyone, everywhere. To achieve this, we need societal infrastructure that enables consumers to make daily choices that support the ideals of veganism. How does that happen? It starts with the development of businesses and organizations that provide vegan products and services. These are businesses that, by their very definition, are built on a foundation of compassion and an ethical standard aimed at creating a better world for everyone. One of the key ideas that I emphasize at Vegan Mainstream is that this vision encompasses all kinds of businesses. When people hear "vegan businesses," it's true that they most often still think of restaurants and other providers of food-related products/ services, but the world's cruelty-free and ethical business needs extend far beyond the food industry.

For the past decade, I have operated my business with the thought that if enough vegans build businesses and align their career choices with their ethics, we will start to see a groundswell of change, and excitingly, that is starting to happen! Of course, not every vegan is going to start a business, but we have seen a definite increase in interest, and I am determined to help as many people go down that path as I can. The other side of the business equation is, of course, the consumer. If consumers understand the difference that vegan businesses make, and they have the opportunity to support vegan businesses, they can also play an important role in advancing the movement—through everyday actions like shopping for vegan grocery items, choosing a vegan financial advisor, eating out at vegan places, hiring a vegan website designer, or buying vegan clothing.

The world is changing. Vegan foods are taking over grocery store shelves, and sustainably sourced materials and zero-waste designs are dominating innovation workshops. Veganism is being embraced in mainstream discussions. However, as every vegan knows, there is still much work to be done. There are disconnects to be reconnected: factory farming must end; climate change must be universally accepted as a fact; and food must nourish us, not harm us.

I believe we can only achieve these things by continuing to build a stable, ethical vegan economy with vibrant workforces and inclusive communities. This is where my dream takes me next. We need money, talent, and scale to fund nonprofit efforts, invest in future businesses, support communities in food deserts, stand up for inequality, and stop the needless suffering of animals.

I'm not the hero of my dream. My role is sometimes major and sometimes minor. Besides, I'm sure I'm not the only one with this particular dream. But the most beautiful part of my dream has been sharing it with others: only by doing this can I make the dream come true.

When I get discouraged, I remember my five-year-old self. If I can dream it, I can make it happen. Once I see the dream, I can start translating it into actionable steps.

Sometimes, one of those steps involves joining an organization like the Jiviniti Coalition to encourage leadership figures like Vice President Kamala Harris to go plant-based for thirty days. Other times, it's taking a leadership role on the VegFund board to support the funding of vegan activism worldwide. It may mean offering my students an extra month of support to help them through an online course. Or simply calling a longtime client to ask how they're doing.

I work hard at my business so I can employ more vegans, help more vegan entrepreneurs, donate more funds to vegan nonprofits, and participate in more activities to make diverse vegan voices heard. My business helps me do my part to realize our vegan future.

Now that I've shared my dream with you, I want to inspire you to envision your vegan dream.

Develop it, act on it, share it, and realize it. I've been running my business for more than ten years now, and while there is always more work to be done, I've seen how the world can change. Every day, my dream helps me live a full, rewarding life that I feel contributes to a better future. It hasn't been easy, but it's always worth it. And now, it's your turn. What does your vision of the future look like and how are you helping to make that a reality?

CLIFTON ROBERTS

Corporate Public Policy Executive, Activist, Speaker

Clifton Roberts was the Humane Party's first-ever presidential candidate and served as the party's staff coordinator for two separate rotations. He is recognized for his visionary, transformational plan for lasting peace, prosperity, and progress for the United States as well as for the world. Representing the rights of all living beings, Roberts is a constitutionalist who believes any country's promise of freedom, peace, and prosperity is deeply rooted in its government's ability to be honest, transparent, innovative, and compassionate. He possesses over twenty-five years of corporate organizational experience in finance, healthcare, and technology and currently serves as a global director of public policy for the foremost data-centric corporation in the world, as part of the company's Governments, Markets, & Trade organization.

THE HEARTS OF NATIONS

My Journey

As a boy, teenager, and young adult, I remember both of my parents used to say to me, "Son, you will never know how I feel until you have children of your own."

In 1995, when I fathered my son, and ten years later, when blessed with a healthy and vegan-conceived baby girl, I finally understood what my mother and father had been telling me over the years. Fatherhood reinvigorated my appreciation of our country. The freedoms it offers. The promise of the pursuit of happiness.

Fatherhood revitalized my appreciation of the founding fathers and the Constitution. My favorite part of the Constitution lives immortally in the Preamble and speaks to the soul of being a parent.

Here, the architects of our commonwealth crafted a clear and concise imperative to "secure the blessings of liberty, to ourselves and our posterity" and, in doing so, ordained our Constitution of the United States of America.

A few years after my son was born, I committed to this imperative by embracing a vegan lifestyle. I had by this time made the connection between the devastating effects of animal agriculture and the broader culture of violence as well as the destruction of our air, land, and water resources. It was a personal choice, as I *awoke* to a vast sea of epiphanies, realizing the importance of my actions for the collective.

Reflections of Our Most Treasured Values

Human rights are protected by our constitutions, which determine our governments' obligations.

Reflecting society's most treasured values, a constitution is an indication of the very heart of a nation. In an ideal world, environmental rights would automatically be included in each and every country's constitution to ensure that every citizen has the right to live in and defend a sound and ecologically balanced environment. Fortunately, ninety countries have included environmental rights in their national constitutions! The guiding principle for such an inclusion declares that human beings have the basic right to live and work in a healthy environment. Consider, if you will, the words of Rachel Carson (author of *Silent Spring*) who, in 1962, said:

> If the Bill of Rights contains no guarantees that a citizen shall be secure against lethal poisons distributed either by private individuals or by public officials, it is surely only because our forefathers, despite their considerable wisdom and foresight, could conceive of no such problem.[8]

Progress and the Long Road Ahead

In 1972, a group of world leaders convened at a groundbreaking global eco-summit, which produced the Stockholm Declaration. The key message established here was that:

Man has the fundamental right to freedom, equality and adequate conditions of life, in an environment of a quality that permits a life of dignity and well-being, and he bears a solemn responsibility to protect and improve the environment for present and future generations.

In the years since the Stockholm Declaration, 177 of the UN's 193 member countries have acknowledged this important right in their own constitutions, international agreements, environmental legislation, and court decisions. Contrarily, countries such as China, Canada, and the United States have yet to do so at a government level. However, it is gratifying to note that various subnational governments have recognized the right to live in a healthy environment. For example, six US states as well as five Canadian provinces and territories have made progress in this area. Nonetheless, we still have a long way to go.

Consent and Dissent

Many people are at opposing ends of the field when it comes to debating the benefits of constitutional environmental rights. Advocates of such an implementation argue that adding environmental rights into their constitutions would enable tougher environmental laws and policies, as well as better implementation and enforcement thereof. Citizens would be encouraged to participate in decision-making involving their environment and would feel accountable, and there would be fewer environmental injustices. In addition, this right would exist in parallel with economic and social rights, and the environment would fare better in the long run. People against the integration of environmental rights into their constitutions believe that such rights would be too vague to be of any use. Given existing environmental laws and human rights, they would be redundant. In addition, they would cause too much litigation and would be difficult to enforce.

Is the constitutional right to live in a healthy environment merely an impossible dream—a whisper with few practical consequences? Or can this right be a powerful change agent, accelerating progress toward a sustainable future? Perhaps the answer lies in the experiences of the ninety-two countries whose citizens already enjoy environmental rights as part of their constitutions. Recent research has revealed that when a country has the right to a healthy environment embedded in its constitution, there are significant legal outcomes, including tougher environmental laws as well as court decisions that defend environmental rights against violations.

Although the US is recognized as a world leader in green, sustainable, and environmental technologies and policies, it benefits our posterity—and ourselves now—for us to remain humble as we evolve as a nation, to evolve while learning from the triumphs and losses of other nations. For evidence substantiates that the benefits prophesied by people just like you and me with a vested interest in green policy and constitutional environmental rights are being realized, while the conceived disadvantages are not occurring.

In some nations, the constitutional right to *greenism*, sustainable and healthy living practices, and environmental protection has become a catalyst for unity and open collaboration. For example, in Argentina, the constitution was reformed in 1994 to incorporate the right to a healthy environment. This had a positive domino effect because many provincial constitutions were then modified to include that right as well. The constitutional right to a healthy environment has also had a significant impact in other countries such as South Africa, Brazil, Costa Rica, Portugal, the Philippines, and Colombia. In addition, we are also witnessing French environmental laws undergoing a similarly positive transformation as a result of the Charter for the Environment of 2005.

In the US, science and politics compete with each other. Scientists are objective, gathering information and utilizing scientific methods in their work. The work of scientists often requires additional time for experimentation and can easily be integrated into public policy. Politicians, by contrast, are led by various factors such as uncertainty, pressure from interest groups, and electoral considerations. Politicians, needing answers before the next election, are also likely to view environmental issues as fraught with idealism. Our government and the citizens elected to represent you and me should reverse this paradigm so that science and politics may coexist. Politics should be free from subjectivity, special interest, ideology, and partisanship.

What We Need

We desperately need a government that is committed to forging a green national identity and that prizes empowered voters like you and me above elite insiders. A government that embraces respect rather than exploitation and initiative rather than entitlement, one that encourages restraint not indulgence, and conservation not waste. We need a regime dedicated to taking an ethical and practical path to avoiding unsustainable and destructive practices that weaken our economy, accelerate our healthcare costs, compromise the future of our posterity, squander our natural resources, engender hostility among our fellow nations, and endanger our national security.

What our country needs is a government committed to ending the use of toxic, hazardous fuels and energy production methods, and replacing them with alternatives that serve the nation's immediate and long-term economic interests. Our government should see no politics in defending our nation's—and the earth's—air, land, and water resources against further contamination and depletion.

We require government representatives who can illustrate—on demand—their commitment to the prevention of anthropogenic effects on air quality, soil quality, and water quality beyond what directly impacts us humans.

We are in need of a government that is unwavering in its effort to preserve the remaining ecosystems of which our nation is a part. This includes protecting all the remaining species of animals who consider these ecosystems home.

Wouldn't it be great if we had a government that understands that in order to revitalize our damaged ecosystems, we must first admit to our role in the root cause of their destruction? Industries such as animal agriculture and dairy farming have been identified as causes of the depletion and contamination of our ozone, soil, and water by global organizations like the United Nations.

We desperately need a government that will protect the rights of all individuals in our country, including nonhuman animals.

And today, we ask that the citizens under this government encourage and empower others within their spheres of influence to commit to the same values. *Green* values.

Call to Action

Spend time to really learn about the elected officials who represent you. I challenge you to research their current representations. Ask yourself questions like, "What are the personal and business interests of my senators and representatives?" or, "Is this person going to represent my green values?" For example, prior to accepting a volunteer officer role with the Humane Party, I signed an oath to live my life—to the best of my ability—according to humane and environmentally considerate principles and values.

Finally, I encourage you to participate in personal activism by educating others about the value of making ethical life choices regarding food, clothing, and politics. This type of activism requires a unique bravery, as those of us who take part in personal activism often do so alone. Fully embracing a humane and compassionate lifestyle remains the most effective way to advocate for environmental rights as well as for the rights of those individuals who are killed in the millions every day in our country and around the world. Humane values provide that all human beings are obligated to serve as responsible stewards of the environment.

In closing, I would like to leave you with a few words from Carl Sagan's book *Pale Blue Dot: A Vision of the Human Future in Space*. This should inspire you all to contemplate the fragility of our precious planet and how we, as women and men, are duty-bound to protect it:

> Look again at that dot. That's here. That's home. That's us. On it everyone you love, everyone you know, everyone you ever heard of, every human being who ever was, lived out their lives. The aggregate of our joy and suffering, thousands of confident

religions, ideologies, and economic doctrines, every hunter and forager, every hero and coward, every creator and destroyer of civilization, every king and peasant, every young couple in love, every mother and father, hopeful child, inventor and explorer, every teacher of morals, every corrupt politician, every "superstar," every "supreme leader," every saint and sinner in the history of our species lived there—on a mote of dust suspended in a sunbeam.[9]

LIN SILVAN

*Animal Lover and Executive Director, Eugene Veg
Education Network (EVEN)*

Lin Silvan spent her professional career in organization development, employee relations, manpower planning, and corporate training for several Fortune 500 companies. She has a BS degree in education, has earned many accolades in business, and is the recipient of the highest professional certifications available in her field. She is also a certified foster parent, a fifty-year member of **MENSA**, and a master gardener with a passion for nature. Lin is an advocate for the animals she loves, the earth she honors, and the vegan movement to which she is dedicated. In 2005, she founded the Eugene Veg Education Network (EVEN). She enjoys spending quality time with her husband Robert, her EVEN co-founder and webmaster, and any canine who follows her home.

BEYOND JOY

Hindsight, they say, is 20/20. And that's a very good thing. What better tool could we use to know what to approach, what to avoid? In the face of our past, hindsight lets us think fresh and decide anew. That clarity surfacing from hindsight urges us to make better choices if we want better results. One of my hindsights was illuminating and painful but quite joyous, as joy comes in many forms.

I was the baby-boomer daughter of Depression-era parents who were generous, kind, and hardworking. I was taught to eat the food put in front of me and to appreciate it because there were "starving children in the world." I never inquired further about where the food came from (the supermarket, right?) or how it got onto my plate (Dad paid for it and Mom cooked it, yes?), and my reality was that loving parents provided, grateful children gave thanks, and I never went to bed hungry. I was too young to know I could inquire, and by the time I was older, I was already on life's journey—in the throes of routines and ruts and those grooves and grinds that would envelop me for decades to come.

Not questioning something as fundamental as food lasted into my forties! As I was preoccupied with school and play, marriage and career, the door just never opened wide enough for the crucial questions. We are all conditioned so that we simply don't ask the incisive questions. However, asking is a learned behavior that just takes practice. Now, in hindsight, I see why I didn't ask. That's why hindsight is such a useful floodlight.

Ask anyone and they will likely tell you they love animals. Dogs and cats always make their list, but farmed animals—the most exploited, who suffer the greatest abuse—remain invisible and are routinely dismissed. We live out our days with total disregard for their circumstances. That's what I did. Oblivious, I chose not to ask, not to see. Sure, I loved animals, but I didn't question their pain, didn't scrutinize their plight, didn't hear their screams. *Yet I would always say I loved animals.* Fortunately, I learned that when you are fully engaged in the love process, you *do* question. So if we love them, why are we complicit in their torment just to appease our polluted palates? After all, that burger or that chicken wing was someone who wanted to live—just like you or me. Not able to speak for themselves, animals resort to screaming and trying to run away as their only hope. Don't we know in our heart of hearts how wrong it all is, especially since it is not necessary? Where are the honor and protection they deserve?

My husband Robert and I took a look inside an animal factory, and our lives were forever changed. The sights, the smells, the shrieks. . . . The overall tenor of a slaughterhouse was a shock to my reality, one that I'll never forget and from which I'll never recover. Once we understood where meat came from, we didn't want it anymore. We didn't want to participate in the horror. We were determined to use the clarity of this new insight to jettison all the cruelty from our diets. We not only don't need meat and dairy to survive, we've been thriving without them. Another good thing about hindsight.

Being vegan is a multifaceted joy—it has health benefits and addresses animal rights concerns as well as environmental and world hunger issues. You can accomplish a lot in a short amount of time as a vegan, and the numerous rewards include a higher quality of life for everyone. As they say, you can sleep better knowing your dinner didn't die screaming.

Being vegan is also a privilege. We work to be a voice on behalf of the animals, because they need all the help they can get. In hindsight, we see that the value of a higher sense of integrity stems from developing a deeper sense of compassion.

Robert and I took our fundamental values and blended them with our sincere desire to give back and help others the way so many had helped and inspired us. We founded the Eugene Veg Education Network (EVEN), a grassroots effort designed to raise awareness, offer inspiration, and provide resources to those wanting to transition to a kinder, healthier lifestyle. Focused on education and outreach, EVEN has been in the trenches for decades, guiding tens of thousands of people. It is not very glamorous, but it is effective—and joyful.

With relevant facts and a clear understanding, we can reflect resolve in our choices. It becomes super easy to muscle through the lies sent out by the meat and dairy industries. There are no difficult or controversial waters when you have all the vital information. To learn: read, read, read. Then peer inside a factory farm. What good is it to know everything if you understand nothing? Apart from all that, there is good news! Once we recognize that these atrocities are being committed on our behalf, there's a lightbulb moment, after which you can't unsee what you saw! You can't unring the chime. Life is not just about you anymore.

Isn't it funny how life is eternally dynamic? Yet most of us only walk (or limp) toward change, and even then, only when forced or persuaded. Change has been known to send even the best people into paralysis. "I love being outside my comfort zone," said no one ever. But what if the change has many benefits?

I understand it is only natural to feel crushed in today's world when we are so frequently beset by disappointment, sorrow, crisis, and betrayal. We miss countless opportunities that come our way that could reinvigorate us with experiences that only the path of compassion can bestow. Persian poet Rumi said: "There is a voice that doesn't use words. Listen." When our thinking is clouded and shallow, and we are too self-absorbed to consider anyone else, travesties happen—and persist. We are complicit in them. I've often wondered why we are always protesting for our rights. Might we march instead, just once, for our responsibilities? What would be a solid plan? Is it time for rethinking? Each of us tends to overlook two very important things. First, how much *choice* we have in doing the things we do, and second, what a huge *impact* even our smallest choice makes! The former will liberate you and the latter will amaze you.

We could talk about the ethos of veganism long into next year, but suffice it to say that we could draw a more humane line. Edgar's Mission Farm Sanctuary says, "If we could live happy and healthy lives without harming others . . . why wouldn't we?" We all possess the power of a noble heart and the strength of an invincible spirit. We can make choices that enrich the world or, at the very least, don't make it worse. Strength is found in learning the truth and breaking free of illusions. Let's not allow our karmic bandits to get the best of us, just because they are familiar.

Any time is a good time to become vegan. Just gather new information from reliable sources, get over any skepticism, and redirect your thinking toward the greater good. Don't be skewed by long-term habits and knee-jerk resistance. It's okay not to be perfect, as long as we allow compassion to continuously move us forward to better decisions. New understandings may be scary at first, but they are powerful and unrelenting—and, yes, joyful! It's exciting to be the revisionist of one's own life. Whose life are we better able to revise than our own? It's been said that "the difference between who you are and who you want to be is what you do." Whenever we see things and think to ourselves, "Someone should do something about that," why not *be* that someone? Step up and do it.

Many waves flow around us, sending us into different phases of our lives. Sometimes, they throw us a little off balance, but they keep us from getting stuck in one spot for too long. It is amazing to watch our actions become habits and our habits become patterns until one day—*voilà!* A new lifestyle. And don't believe the hype! Being vegan is extremely easy. There is great joy in doing things right and greater joy in doing the right things.

Never before has there been more meaningful and precise vegan information available to everyone. Books, blogs, and videos. Food, recipes, nutrition studies. Veganism is a swift-moving current, and there is no need to hold on to the riverbank. Easy, simple information is accessible to the masses to make the changes needed for a better world— for the animals, for the planet, and for the people. We simply need to see clearly to get our lives right. A whole-food, plant-based diet just keeps delivering extraordinary results for everyone.

The future is beyond bright, and it is easy to be optimistic in light of major positivity and change. Veganism has been gaining momentum and now has a stronghold everywhere in the mainstream. Food, clothing, cosmetics, cruise lines, airlines, restaurants. . . . The greatly underestimated US$15 billion vegan food industry alone is headed to over US$71 billion in the next several years. Its growth being intertwined with advances in other, related industries, and since veganism right now has great velocity, I believe that is a conservative number.

EVEN was established as a grassroots group based in Eugene, Oregon, but has grown over 11,000 percent in just the past decade. The kids say the growth of veganism is "way cool," and surely, this is because it is not just a trend, a newfangled fad, or a pet rock craze. We hear from folks around the world, because veganism is a long-overdue, liberating, and massive groundswell that brings hope and joy with it. The world's problems can never be solved by the darkness that produced them. In a world of darkness, veganism is a beacon of light.

French writer Victor Hugo said that there is nothing more powerful than an idea whose time has come. Veganism is that idea, and *that* is beyond joyful!

KRISSI VANDENBERG

Executive Director, Vegan Action

Krissi Vandenberg became an ethical vegan in 1995, inspired by friends and the British cookzine *Soy Not Oi!* She began as a volunteer for Vegan Action in Berkeley, California, in 1998 and has served as executive director since bringing the organization to Richmond, Virginia, in 2000. She co-founded the Richmond Animal Rights Network. Krissi has a Bachelor of Science in biology, a Master of Science in sociology, and a certificate in nonprofit management, all from Virginia Commonwealth University. She has presented on vegan-related issues at festivals around the country and was a top presenter at the 2015 Nonprofit Learning Point Summit. Krissi is also passionate about feminism, human rights, and nature and the environment; she is a Certified Tree Steward.

POSITIVE ACTIVISM FOR LIFELONG CHANGE

I grew up like most folks in the US, eating meat and eggs and drinking milk. I've been a serious animal lover from a young age, and I remember having a hard time eating some animal products—specifically the ones I could tell came from an identifiable animal, such as chicken legs, pork chops, and ribs. But I still ate the standard food because it was provided for me, it was modeled as normal, and I was told it was healthy. Everything around me said that I should ignore my feelings, that my instincts of kindness and concern should not apply to my food. Over the years, that is what I did. Like most of us, I continued to eat animals but espoused a love for cats and dogs. Everything in my environment and my culture told me it was acceptable and right to eat some animals while loving others.

Approximately eighty billion animals are killed every year for food in the cruelest ways you could imagine. Animal waste from factory farms is among the greatest pollutants of our waterways in the US. The demand for livestock pasture is a major driver of deforestation. We have a hunger epidemic in our country; some children are eating just one meal a day or not at all. We are growing the majority of grain, corn, and soy to feed other animals to then feed people. We could be feeding people with these grains, but we are feeding them to animals instead. It's illogical and inefficient. The earth is warming every year at an unprecedented rate. Sea levels are rising; the global temperature is rising. Arctic sea ice is declining; glaciers are retreating; and oceans are becoming more acidic. The scientific consensus is that the increase of carbon dioxide in our atmosphere is due to human activity. Our choices, our behaviors, and our beliefs are all contributing to the decline in the health of our planet and to the unnecessary suffering of others.

These issues spoke to me in my freshman year of college. Once I learned about all of the violence involved in raising animals for food and that there is no reason or requirement to eat animals to thrive and be healthy, I recognized that what I'd been doing was absolutely antithetical to my aspiration to be as compassionate as possible. I had an epiphany—I could not continue to eat animals while being so concerned for them, the environment, and the wellbeing of other people on this planet, so I decided to be vegan. Once I had made that transition, I realized that I wasn't going to be able to save every single animal, but I wanted to make sure that I was making choices and decisions every day in my life to do the very best I could. I wanted to strive to live as compassionately as possible and to share that information with other people so they could do the very same.

So I got involved in local activism for animal rights, human rights, and environmental protection. Getting active gave me meaning and fulfillment, and I urgently wanted to convince as many people as possible to care about these issues. That was much easier said than done; it just wasn't happening, and I was miserable and angry. I was angry that everyone didn't see what I saw that was broken in the world. I was angry that people weren't up in arms about the mistreatment of animals and the condition of the earth and weren't doing everything in their power to change things for the better. I constantly talked about how terrible things were in the world; I reminded people about the billions of animals killed for food every year, about the rainforest land cut down to raise those animals, about the pollutants released into our waterways from factory farms, and about the millions of people suffering from hunger. I was determined to get through to people no matter what it took—evoking guilt, anger, or extreme sadness.

While these strategies seemed to strike a chord with people, they also seemed to scare them away from action, not drive them to it. I was focusing on yelling at people, harassing people, showing graphic photos, and various other guilt-inducing tactics that would get attention. While I was feeling justified in expressing my frustration with these injustices in the world, I was not inducing change. Most people would just shut down or walk away. I was not encouraging or inspiring people to see the issues and act. They admitted they wanted to see change, to see the world become a better place, but they just would not take the steps to change their own behaviors and themselves. I was starting to see those who would not change as lazy, uncaring, unmotivated, or willfully ignorant.

I was driven by anger, and I eventually realized that this was not sustainable. In addition to constantly feeling overwhelmed myself, I also realized I was overwhelming everyone around me. Guilt, sadness, and anger may have an immediate impact that results in behavioral change in some, but this change often does not last. The lesson I needed to learn is that the future of changemaking lies in the positive, purposeful, and inspirational motivation of others, through modeling positive change. Positive change by positive means is the ultimate success. It means helping people make a change by choice, for the right reasons that speak to them. It is our duty as activists to help people find those reasons.

When people make a change for the better, for reasons that mean something to them, they are more likely to stick with that decision and, even better, influence others to change. This form of activism, aimed at influencing both collective behavior and social action, is both fulfilling and sustainable; over time, it leads to the long-term involvement of and positive impact created by more and more people.

Some people say that either a person has the drive to change or they don't. But I don't believe that. Everyone has the ability; they just have to choose to use it. All the time, we are bombarded with terrible things happening all over the world. We often have to look the other way just to keep going and living. It is hard to address issues revolving around suffering; it takes strength and courage to face them. It is not easy to choose to make a lifestyle change. But you know what they say about the path of least resistance: there's nothing worthwhile at the end.

The future of change is right in front of us. The key is finding and seeing the good in others, seeing the positive impacts we each are having in our communities and on the planet. Today, I don't forget about the state of the planet—what is happening to the animals, the trees, the people, and our natural resources. But I also see more and more people choosing a plant-based diet for the animals, for their health, for the environment, for global food security; more and more people donating their time, money, and resources to improve their communities; and more and more people changing their behaviors to better the environment. People are beginning to examine their behaviors and themselves and are making better choices for the planet. More people are actively making the effort to not eat animals and animal products, to buy local products, support local companies, improve our environment, and appreciate and take care of the resources we have.

I am fortunate to have been able to focus on my passions—animals and the environment—and I have the honor of serving as the director of Vegan Action, where we work to encourage people to choose a plant-based diet for the benefit of the animals, the environment, and us humans. We encourage people to make the best decisions they can, to vote with their dollars every day, in everything they do. We work to provide as many resources as possible—to reach the greatest number of people and to inspire them to choose vegan as often as they can. Remember, whatever we demand will continue to be supplied. I find myself saying things I judged people for saying to me when I was a new vegan in my early twenties. Now, they ring true. I remind people that we have more strength and effect more change by being kind and open, even when that is very hard to do. Even when we feel anger and hatred toward what is happening to the animals and the earth, I believe we will bring out true change by influencing people to make positive choices, which last much longer than do the choices people make out of guilt or fear. I know it is ideological, but I want people to change for the right reasons.

Why should you care? Because we are all in this together, and we all share this space. And don't we all want to do things that matter in life? So how do we start working toward collective change? I believe it's truly about inspiring others in our everyday lives to change; it's all in how we treat other people, how we respect others' beliefs, how we live our lives, how we volunteer our time and give back to our community. Honestly, most often, change takes place one person and one day at a time. Things will keep getting worse if we don't start trying to make them better. We cannot hope that things will change; we can't wait for someone else to make a change. It's up to each one of us, but we don't have to do it alone. Let's create some positive change together!

AFTERWORD

Dr. Joanne Kong

As I reflect upon the essays in this book, it is clear to me that fundamental changes are vital as humankind moves forward from present-day challenges and threats, which are unprecedented in our lifetimes and the seriousness of which cannot be denied, whether they are related to the coronavirus, climate change and environmental devastation, food injustice, world hunger, poverty, disease, or rising social inequities. In the face of these seemingly insurmountable problems, we can easily feel powerless, as if there were little we as individuals could do to make a difference.

Yet, as so eloquently presented throughout this book, the guiding paths to change can be found within. Crafting our lives with heartfelt intention and aligning our actions with our values can be sources of tremendous transformative power. Even if the essential aspects of human nature might not change, it is through widening our perspectives, insights, and ways of thinking that we can envision new directions for how we live that are grounded in a higher level of caring and kinship.

We can dare to question the underlying societal beliefs and customs that have been accepted as concrete, unchangeable realities. We can open our eyes to what we have been conditioned *not* to see—the horrific cruelties committed with massive indifference against innocent sentient beings, acts we would never wish upon ourselves or others. It is long past the time to question an industry that has distanced and numbed us from our deep capacities for empathy and compassion. We must also question a society that is dominated by self-interest and limitless material gain and that is wreaking destruction on the planet as if its resources were inexhaustible and meant solely for our short-term use. Our mandate must be nothing less than a broadscale intervention for the health of the planet.

Veganism is growing around the world; the diversity of countries represented in this book shows the growing global awareness of the benefits of a plant-based lifestyle. A new sense of identity will emerge out of our collective efforts to create a kinder and more sustainable world—one that says we are *one* global family, *one* world consciousness bound together by our shared humanity. In that process, veganism becomes a vehicle to celebrate the things that connect us. It is not a movement restricted to the interests of a particular group based on social class, economic status, race, or gender; it is rooted in the commonalities shared by all living beings, among them the desire to live free from pain and suffering, to have adequate nourishment and shelter, to communicate and socialize, and to protect our young. We all seek companionship; we love one another, feel joy and sadness; and if necessary, we will fight for our lives.

We must allow ourselves to be bold in the hope that we *will* see a vegan world in the near future; in fact, we should be of the mindset that it has already arrived. One need only point to the signs that veganism has already moved into the mainstream: the astounding explosion of the plant-based food industry in recent years as well as the availability of other cruelty-free products, rising activism for animal rights around the world, the increased presence of the vegan message on social media and the Internet, and the development of new food technologies and agricultural practices to promote healthy and sustainable sources of nutrition for a growing world population.

Our mission to create and nurture a more compassionate world is best achieved when we realize that opening ourselves to new possibilities in our lives is *not* about restriction, loss, or deprivation. If anything, it's the opposite. To let go of food habits and beliefs that are not only harmful to our health but also result in unimaginable cruelty exacted upon animals is an act of great liberation. It's about removing the inner conflict—the cognitive dissonance—of enabling violence on a massive scale and at the same time professing to love animals. It's about embracing compassion through one of the most basic aspects of our everyday lives—what we choose to eat. And it's about gaining a sense of equanimity in our emotional lives, for in making the choice to nourish our bodies with the positive energy of plant foods, our inner beings can begin to overflow with peace, kindness, and mindfulness. To me, these are some of the greatest gifts of being vegan. I can't tell you how many times I have met people who, while they had initially gone plant-based for (mostly) health or environmental reasons, saw their ethical convictions grow naturally, along with the realization that veganism is connected to the deep awareness that we are all a part of the same life energy.

In making lifestyle choices that will determine our shared destiny, we can embrace the idea that every individual *does* make a difference. I've often wondered about the energies that make up our lives, the essence of what it means to be conscious and sentient. While the ability to explain all the mysteries of life certainly lies beyond our reach, we do know this: all of our actions and everything that we think and feel become manifest in the world around us.

I look into the future and see the possibilities for a bold new world brought about by the best qualities of who we are—our intellect, adaptability, sense of innovation, perseverance, optimism, and determination. We end the ravages upon our planet, instead regenerating and preserving its resources that allow us to live; we find strength in our diversity; we continue to recognize and accept the emotional and cognitive abilities of nonhuman animals; and we expand the rising awareness that food should be healing and not come from violence. I believe that one day, we will look back upon the mass exploitation of animals as a moral atrocity. Bringing it to an end will be proof of a revolutionary kindness and one of humanity's greatest acts of compassion.

NOTES

SECTION ONE: Our Kindred Animals

1. The Associated Press, "Graphic Abuse of Pigs Caught on Tape," *CBS News*, September 17, 2008, https://www.cbsnews.com/news/graphic-abuse-of-pigs-caught-on-tape/; The Associated Press, "Undercover Video Shows Workers Abusing Pigs," *NBC News*, September 17, 2008, http://www.nbcnews.com/id/26757660/ns/us_news-crime_and_courts/t/undercover-video-shows-workers-abusing-pigs/; PETA, "Mother Pigs and Piglets Abused by Hormel Supplier," PETA Investigations, September 2008, http://investigations.peta.org/mother-pigs-piglets-abused-hormel-supplier/.

2. "Investigator 1 Log Notes—IA Sow Farm" (notes, outside Bayard, IA, 2008), https://assets.documentcloud.org/documents/1314070/investigator-1-log-notes.pdf; "Investigator 2 Log Notes—IA Sow Farm" (notes, outside Bayard, IA, 2008), https://assets.documentcloud.org/documents/1314069/investigator-2-log-notes.pdf.

3. "Animals Are Not Ours to Eat," Annual Report 2008, PETA, 2009, https://web.archive.org/web/20090514042532/http://www.peta.org/feat/annual review/notToEat.asp.

4. Associated Press, "Undercover Video Shows Workers Abusing Pigs"; Associated Press, "Graphic Abuse of Pigs Caught on Tape."

5. National Pork Board and American Association of Swine Veterinarians, "On Farm Euthanasia of Swine—Options for the Producer," last revised 2016, https://www.aasv.org/aasv/euthanasia.pdf; Gail Golab and American Veterinary Medical Association, "Hot on Facebook: Euthanasia of Suckling Pigs Using Blunt Force Trauma," AVMA Work Blog, July 21, 2012, http://atwork.avma.org/2012/07/21/hot-on-facebook-euthanasia-of-suckling-pigs-using-blunt-force-trauma/; Steven L. Leary and American Veterinary Medical Association, *AVMA Guidelines for the Euthanasia of Animals: 2013 Edition*, 2013, https://www.avma.org/KB/Policies/Documents/euthanasia.pdf.

6. "Blunt Force Trauma Ensures Humane Pig Euthanasia, Says Veterinary Council," The Pig Site, October 25, 2016, http://www.thepigsite.com/swinenews/42569/blunt-force-trauma-ensures-humane-pig-euthanasia-says-veterinary-council/; Emily Moran Barwick, "Do Animals Want to Be Eaten?" Bite Size Vegan, May 16, 2016, http://www.bitesizevegan.org/bite-size-vegan-nuggets/main-nuggets/do-animals-want-to-be-eaten/.

7. "Council Regulation (EC) No 1099/2009 of 24 September 2009 on the Protection of Animals at the Time of Killing," *Official Journal of the European Union*, L 303 (2009): 1–30, https://eur-lex.europa.eu/eli/reg/2009/1099/oj.

8. *Animal Welfare: Issues and Opportunities in the Meat, Poultry, and Egg Markets in the U.S.* (market research report, *Packaged Facts*, April 10, 2017), https://www.packagedfacts.com/Animal-Welfare-Meat-10771767/.

9. *Study on Information to Consumers on the Stunning of Animals: Final Report* (Brussels: European Commission, February 23, 2015), http://ec.europa.eu/food/animals/docs/aw_practice_slaughter_fci-stunning_report_en.pdf; Safefood, "Where Does Our Food Come From?" (consumer-focused review, Safefood, July 2009), http://www.safefood.eu/SafeFood/media/SafeFoodLibrary/Documents/Publications/Market%20Research/Safefood_Food-Origin_CFR.pdf; "Farm Animal Welfare," American Society for the Prevention of Cruelty to Animals, accessed October 3, 2018, https://www.aspca.org/animal-cruelty/farm-animal-welfare; "Consumer Perceptions of Farm Animal Welfare," Animal Welfare Institute, accessed November 17, 2020, https://awionline.org/sites/default/files/uploads/documents/fa-consumer_perceptionsoffarmwelfare_-112511.pdf; Susan Kelly, "Millennials Drive Rise in Fresh-Meat Buying: Study," *New Mexico Stockman*, June 2018; Consumer Reports, "Food Labels Survey," (survey research report, Consumer Reports National Research Center, 2014); Lake Research Partners, "Farm Animal Research Survey Findings," ASPCA, accessed November 17, 2020, https://www.aspca.org/sites/default/files/aspca_2012_aggag_survey.pdf; Lake Research Partners, "Animal Welfare Labeling," Online Survey Public Memo (online survey public memo, ASPCA, February 1, 2019), https://www.aspca.org/sites/default/files/aspca-2018_animal_welfare_labelling_and_consumer_concern_survey.pdf; "Label Confusion: How 'Humane' and 'Sustainable' Claims on Meat Packages Deceive Consumers" (Animal Welfare Institute, January 19, 2017), https://awionline.org/sites/default/files/publication/digital_download/19LabelConfusionReport.pdf.

10. "Study on Information to Consumers on the Stunning of Animals: Final Report"; Safefood, "Where Does Our Food Come From?"; "Consumer Perceptions of Farm Animal Welfare"; Kelly, "Millennials Drive Rise in Fresh-Meat Buying: Study"; Consumer Reports, "Food Labels Survey"; "Buying Meat" (survey, YouGov, 2018), https://today.yougov.com/topics/food/articles-reports/2018/11/26/ethical-meat-price-quality-animal-rights.

11. "Treaty of Lisbon Amending the Treaty on European Union and the Treaty Establishing the European Community, Signed at Lisbon, 13 December 2007," *Official Journal of the European Union*, C 306 (2009): 1–271; "The Treaty of Lisbon: Introduction," EUR-Lex, accessed September 4, 2016.

12. "Council Regulation (EC) No 1099/2009 of 24 September 2009 on the Protection of Animals at the Time of Killing."

13. "Farmed Animals and the Law," Animal Legal Defense Fund, accessed November 6, 2016, http://aldf.org/resources/advocating-for-animals/farmed-animals-and-the-law/; "Farm Animal Welfare"; "Government Regulation of Factory Farms," The National Humane Education Society, accessed October 3, 2018, https://nhes.org/3372-2/.

14. *The Animal Welfare Act*, Public Law 89–544, *U.S. Code* 7 (1966), https://www.nal.usda.gov/awic/animal-welfare-act; "Animal Welfare Act History Digital Collection," Animal Welfare Act History Digital Collection, US Department of Agriculture, accessed October 15, 2019, https://awahistory.nal.usda.gov/; Animal and Plant Health Inspection Service and United States Department of Agriculture, "Animal Welfare Act and Animal Welfare Regulations," July 2020, https://www.aphis.usda.gov/animal_welfare/downloads/bluebook-ac-awa.pdf; "Transportation, Sale, and Handling of Certain Animals," Public Law 89–544, *U.S. Code* 7 (1966), https://www.law.cornell.edu/uscode/text/7/chapter-54.

15. "Farmed Animals and the Law"; "Farm Animal Welfare."

16. "Council Regulation (EC) No 1099/2009 of 24 September 2009 on the protection of animals at the time of killing." Within the finalized legislation, see the fourth row of "Table 1—Mechanical methods" in "Chapter I—Methods" of Annex 1, and see further specifications under "2. Maceration" in "Chapter II—Specific requirements for certain methods" of Annex 1.

17. *Commission Staff Working Document Accompanying the Proposal for a Council Regulation on the Protection of Animals at the Time of Killing: Impact Assessment Report* (Brussels: Commission of the European Communities, 2008).

18. "Project In Ovo—Animal Welfare & Efficiency," Project In Ovo, accessed September 1, 2016, https://web.archive.org/web/20160617073856/http://project.inovo.nl:80/.

19. *Commission Staff Working Document Accompanying the Proposal for a Council Regulation on the Protection of Animals at the Time of Killing: Impact Assessment Report.*

20. Coalition for Sustainable Egg Supply, "Final Research Results Report," Laying Hen Housing Research Project (The Center for Food Integrity, 2015), https://www2.sustainableeggcoalition.org/final-results.

21. United States Department of Agriculture, "Free Range or Free Roaming," in *Meat and Poultry Labeling Terms*, accessed November 23, 2020, https://www.fsis.usda.gov/food-safety/safe-food-handling-and-preparation/food-safety-basics/meat-and-poultry-labeling-terms.

22. "Dangerous Contaminated Chicken: Confusing Chicken Labels Decoded," *Consumer Reports*, January 2014, https://www.consumerreports.org/cro/magazine/2014/02/the-high-cost-of-cheap-chicken/index.htm.

23. "Label Confusion: How 'Humane' and 'Sustainable' Claims on Meat Packages Deceive Consumers."

24. Food Safety and Inspection Service, "Food Safety and Inspection Service Labeling Guideline on Documentation Needed to Substantiate Animal Raising Claims for Label Submissions" (United States Department of Agriculture, December 2019).

25. Statistics Division (ESS), "FAOSTAT: Livestock Primary," Food and Agriculture Organization of the United Nations, accessed May 11, 2015.

26. "Council Directive 1999/74/EC of 19 July 1999 Laying down Minimum Standards for the Protection of Laying Hens," *Official Journal of the European Communities*, L 203 (1999): 53–57.

27. "Animal Welfare: Commission Urges 13 Member States to Implement Ban on Laying Hen Cages," European Commission, January 26, 2012, http://europa.eu/rapid/press-release_IP-12-47_en.htm?locale=en.

28. "Animal Welfare: Commission Increases Pressure on Member States to Enforce Group Housing of Sows," European Commission, February 21, 2013, http://europa.eu/rapid/press-release_IP-13-135_en.htm; "Government of Ireland, "S.I. No. 91/1995 - European Communities (Welfare of Pigs) Regulations, 1995." (1995), http://www.irishstatutebook.ie/eli/1995/si/91/made/en/print; Council of the EU, "Council Directive 2001/88/EC of 23 October 2001 Amending Directive 91/630/EEC Laying Down Minimum Standards for the Protection of Pigs," *2011*/88/EC § (2001); "Council Directive 2008/120/EC of 18 December 2008 Laying down Minimum Standards for the Protection of Pigs (Codified Version)," *Official Journal of the European Union*, L 47 (2009): 5–13. The non-compliant member states were Belgium, Cyprus, Denmark, France, Germany, Greece, Ireland, Poland, and Portugal.

29. "Animal Protection Index," World Animal Protection, 2014, http://api.worldanimalprotection.org/; Cecilia Mille and Eva Frejadotter Diesen, *The Best Animal Welfare in the World? An Investigation into the Myth about Sweden*, trans. Niki Woods (Djurens Rätt, 2009), http://www.djurensratt.se/sites/default/files/best-animal-welfare-in-the-world.pdf. Regarding the thirteen member states that failed to implement the battery cage ban: The Netherlands is one of only five countries to receive the highest rating for animal welfare according to the Animal Protection Index; Spain, France, Italy, and Poland account for half of the countries ranked second highest in animal welfare. Regarding countries that failed to implement the gestation crate ban: Denmark is one of only five countries to receive the highest rating for animal welfare according to the Animal Protection Index. France, Germany, and Poland are ranked second highest in animal welfare. France and Poland failed to implement both the battery cage and gestation crate bans. Note that the Animal Protection Index does not currently include all countries. Even the most idealized countries— like Sweden, for example—are far from ideal upon closer inspection.

30. The Humane Society of the United States, "An HSUS Report: The Welfare of Cows in the Dairy Industry," *Agribusiness Reports* 2009, no. 1 (2009), https://www. wellbeingintlstudiesrepository.org/hsus_reps_impacts_on_animals/20/.

31. Colchester and Greenwood, "Chickenomics: How Chicken Became the Rich World's Most Popular Meat," *Economist*, January 19, 2019.

32. Tris Allison, ed., *State of the World's Birds: Taking the Pulse of the Planet* (Cambridge, UK: BirdLife International, 2018), https://www.birdlife.org/ sites/default/files/attachments/BL_ReportENG_V11_spreads.pdf.

33. Rachel Carson, *Silent Spring* (New York: Fawcett Crest, 1962), 97.

34. Brian Owens, "Pharmaceuticals in the Environment: A Growing Problem," *The Pharmaceutical Journal*, 2015, https://pharmaceutical-journal.com/ article/feature/pharmaceuticals-in-the-environment-a-growing-problem.

35. Michael W. Fox, "Animal Freedom and Well-Being: Want or Need?" *Applied Animal Ethology* 11 (1983–4): 205–9.

36. Carson, *Silent Spring*, 114.

37. Emily Dickinson, "'Hope' is the Thing with Feathers," The Poetry Foundation, https://www.poetryfoundation.org/poems/42889/hope-is-the-thing -with-feathers-314.

38. Jonathan Balcombe, "Playing, Courting, and Vanity: The Rich Emotional Lives of Fish," *Plant Based News*, March 13, 2019, https://plantbasednews. org/culture/playing-courting-and-vanity-rich-emotional-lives-fish/.

39. Isaac Bashevis Singer, Aliza Shevrin, and Elizabeth Shub, *Enemies, a Love Story* (New York: Farrar, Straus and Giroux, 1998), 257.

40. Thomas Byron and Ram Dass, "Violence," in *Dhammapada: The Sayings of the Buddha* (Boulder: Shambhala Publications, 1996), 36.

SECTION TWO: Around the Globe

1. Sunny Gandara, "5 Signs That There's a Vegan Takeover Happening in Norway," *VegNews*, January 2, 2019, https://vegnews. com/2019/1/5-signs-that-theres-a-vegan-takeover-happening-in-norway.

2. Dean Best, "Orkla CEO Forecasts Jump in Plant-Based Sales," Just Food, September 18, 2020, https://www.just-food.com/news/orkla-ceo-forecasts-jump-in-plant-based-sales_id144410.aspx.

3. "Animal Protection Index," World Animal Protection, https://api.worldanimalprotection.org/country/japan.

4. Markus Winkler, "Veganism in Japan," Bord Bia – The Irish Food Board, August 10, 2020, https://www.bordbia.ie/industry/news/food-alerts/2020/ veganism-in-japan/.

5. "Number of German Vegans Doubles to 2.6 Million in Just Four Years," *Vegconomist*, November 18, 2020, https://vegconomist.com/

studies-and-numbers/number-of-german-vegans-doubles-to-2-6-million-in-just-four-years/.

6. "European Chicken Commitment," Albert Schweitzer Foundation, https://albertschweitzerfoundation.org/campaigns/european-chicken-commitment.

7. "Announcing Our 2020 Charity Recommendations," Animal Charity Evaluators, November 24, 2020, https://animalcharityevaluators.org/blog/announcing-our-2020-charity-recommendations/.

SECTION THREE: Activism

1. Jillian Sullivan, *Map for the Heart: Ida Valley Essays* (Dunedin, New Zealand: Otago University Press, 2020), 160.

2. Leo Tolstoy, *A Calendar of Wisdom: Daily Thoughts to Nourish the Soul*, trans. Peter Sekirin (New York: Scribner, 1997).

3. Professor Philip Armstrong, head of the Department of English at Canterbury University and member of the Centre for Human–Animal Studies, has written a book about sheep in New Zealand's colonial context: Philip Armstrong, *Sheep* (London: Reaktion, 2016).

4. Tolstoy, *A Calendar of Wisdom*.

5. Eve Ensler, foreword to *My Name Is Jody Williams: A Vermont Girl's Winding Path to the Nobel Peace Prize*, by Jody Williams (Oakland: University of California Press, 2013), ix.

SECTION FOUR: Body and Spirit

1. Rolf Sovik, "Yoga Philosophy Basics: The 5 Yamas," *Yoga International*, accessed November 30, 2020, https://yogainternational.com/article/view/yoga-philosophy-basics-the-5-yamas.

SECTION FIVE: The Arts

1. John Holmes, "Losing 25,000 to Hunger Every Day," *UN Chronicle* 45, no. 3 (December 2009): 14–20.

2. Emily S. Cassidy, Paul C. West, James S. Gerber, and Jonathan A. Foley, "Redefining Agricultural Yields: From Tonnes to People Nourished per Hectare," *Environmental Research Letters* 8, no. 3 (2013).

3. "Frequently Asked Questions on Climate Change and Disaster Displacement," The United Nations Refugee Center, November 6, 2016, www.unhcr.org/news/latest/2016/11/581f52dc4/frequently-asked-questions-climate-change-disaster-displacement.html.

SECTION SIX: A New Future

1. Martin C. Heller and Gregory A. Keoleian, *Beyond Meat's Beyond Burger Life Cycle Assessment: A Detailed Comparison between a Plant-based and an Animal-based Protein Source* (Center for Sustainable Systems, University of Michigan, 2018), http://css.umich.edu/publication/beyond-meats-beyond-burger-life-cycle-assessment-detailed-comparison-between-plant-based.

2. Mike Murphy, "Beyond Meat Soars 163% in Biggest-Popping U.S. IPO since 2000," *MarketWatch*, May 2, 2019, https://www.marketwatch.com/story/beyond-meat-soars-163-in-biggest-popping-us-ipo-since-2000-2019-05-02.

3. "American Dairy Farmers Depend on Government Subsidies," *Markets Insider*, February 8, 2018, https://markets.businessinsider.com/news/stocks/american-dairy-farmers-depend-on-government-subsidies-1015126442.

4. "Paul Chatlin, Founder," Plant Based Nutrition Study Group, accessed November 20, 2020, https://www.pbnsg.org/partner-collection/2015/10/17/paul-chatlin-founder.

5. This compilation is based on Jeremy Lent's comprehensively referenced research work: Jeremy Lent, "The Five Real Conspiracies You Need to Know About," Resilience, October 2, 2020, https://www.resilience.org/stories/2020-10-02/the-five-real-conspiracies-you-need-to-know-about/.

6. These statistics from the US Department of Agriculture were reported by Dr. Michael Greger: Michael Greger, "Where Do You Get Your Fiber?" Nutrition Facts, September 29, 2015, https://nutritionfacts.org/2015/09/29/where-do-you-get-your-fiber/.

7. The *Aquarius* bottom-up money flow system is currently being designed to implement Kate Raworth's *Donut Economics* on the Holochain platform.

8. Rachel Carson, *Silent Spring* (New York: Houghton Mifflin Company, 1962), 12–13.

9. Carl Sagan, *Pale Blue Dot: A Vision of the Human Future in Space* (New York: Random House Publishing Group, 1994), 339–40.

ABOUT THE EDITOR

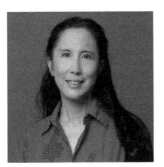 DR. JOANNE KONG speaks around the world as a vegan advocate and is the author of *If You've Ever Loved an Animal, Go Vegan*. She is featured in *Legends of Change*, a collection of stories about vegan women changing the world, and has been praised for her TEDx talk *The Power of Plant-Based Eating* and the video *An Urgent Plea for Healing: Cherish All Animals*. An award-winning classical pianist, she holds a Doctor of Musical Arts degree from the University of Oregon and draws upon a diversity of skills as a writer, speaker, and creative artist in her advocacy activities.

Dr. Kong is currently a faculty member and sustainability advisor at the University of Richmond in Virginia.

ABOUT THE PUBLISHER

LANTERN PUBLISHING & MEDIA was founded in 2020 to follow and expand on the legacy of Lantern Books—a publishing company started in 1999 on the principles of living with a greater depth and commitment to the preservation of the natural world. Like its predecessor, Lantern Publishing & Media produces books on animal advocacy, veganism, religion, social justice, humane education, psychology, family therapy, and recovery. Lantern is dedicated to printing in the United States on recycled paper and saving resources in our day-to-day operations. Our titles are also available as e-books and audiobooks.

To catch up on Lantern's publishing program, visit us at www.lanternpm.org.

 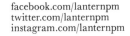

facebook.com/lanternpm
twitter.com/lanternpm
instagram.com/lanternpm